Outcomes of Skin Surgery

Outcomes of Skin Surgery

Graham Colver DM FRCP

Consultant Dermatologist
Chesterfield Royal Hospital
United Kingdom

Former President
British Society for Dermatological Surgery

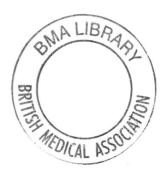
informa
healthcare

©2008 Informa Ltd

First published in the United Kingdom in 2008 by Informa Healthcare, Telephone House, 69–77 Paul Street, London EC2A 4LQ. Informa Healthcare is a trading division of Informa UK Ltd. Registered Office: 37/41 Mortimer Street, London W1T 3JH. Registered in England and Wales number 1072954.

Tel: +44 (0)20 7017 5000
Fax: +44 (0)20 7017 6699
Website: www.informahealthcare.com

A CIP record for this book is available from the British Library.
Library of Congress Cataloging-in-Publication Data

Data available on application

ISBN-10: 0 415 47038 2
ISBN-13: 978 0 415 47038 4

Distributed in North and South America by
Taylor & Francis
6000 Broken Sound Parkway, NW, (Suite 300)
Boca Raton, FL 33487, USA

Within Continental USA
Tel: 1 (800) 272 7737; Fax: 1 (800) 374 3401
Outside Continental USA
Tel: (561) 994 0555; Fax: (561) 361 6018
Email: orders@crcpress.com

Book orders in the rest of the world
Paul Abrahams
Tel: +44 (0)20 7017 4036
Email: bookorders@informa.com

Composition by Exeter Premedia Services Private Ltd., Chennai, India
Printed and bound in India by Replika Press Pvt Ltd

Contents

Acknowledgements

This book has been published on behalf of the British Society for Dermatological Surgery (BSDS), which is affiliated to the British Association of Dermatologists. The BSDS is dedicated to training dermatologists to high standards in all aspects of skin surgery.

Members of the BSDS are busy, in their everyday practice, with surgical and other physical treatments of the skin. The Society is interested in any medium which might help patients to grasp the scope and implications of these treatments and has supported publication of the book. It is hoped that the illustrations of the possible outcomes of skin surgery will improve the process of consent.

I am very grateful to the following members of the BSDS who have contributed to the book:

Dr Catriona Irvine
Dr Graeme Stables
Dr James Langtry
Dr Andrew Affleck

Graham Colver

Introduction

Surgical procedures on the skin are carried out throughout the world and in many settings. They encompass two chief groups, the first of which is disease orientated. It includes procedures such as excision of benign and malignant tumours, diagnostic biopsies, cryosurgery, curettage for superficial lesions and photodynamic therapy. The second group is chiefly cosmetic in approach and includes chemical and laser peels, face lifts, liposuction and fillers.

This book concentrates on the procedures included in the first group and is intended to help people understand the types of outcome that can be expected from different procedures. It is common experience that some people have a neat, flat appendix scar while others might have a raised rather ragged-looking scar. In this case the reasons for a poorer outcome could include a wound infection, exercising too quickly after the operation and an individual's natural healing mechanisms.

It is clear that the results of skin surgery vary considerably between individuals and it is sensible to outline the range of possibilities at the outset. Sometimes the term 'minor surgery' can give the impression that nothing can go wrong but there are side effects and possible complications from the simplest of procedures.

Any practitioner who undertakes procedures has a duty to be properly trained and to have adequate knowledge of all the possible outcomes of treatment. The process of consent involves discussion about the need for treatment and the natural history of the condition without intervention. The treatment options should be enumerated with brief discussion of their relative merits in terms of success and side effects and risks (i.e. the risk–benefit ratio).

The book has intentionally a limited text. It is designed to be shared, with the photographs, between doctors and patients. It highlights the side effects and complications, giving some idea of frequency, if known, and the factors which might increase the chance of a particular event.

No treatment

No treatment might be best – harmless lesions

Doctors are frequently asked if anything needs to be done about a skin lesion or blemish. Often they are harmless and natural and many patients, especially if they are slightly guarded about intervention, willingly take the advice to 'do nothing'.

Offering the 'no treatment option' should always be part of the consultation for benign lesions. Despite the contents of the referral letter from the general practitioner and even the initial expressed wish of the patient it is quite common to discover some misunderstanding about the exact nature of the lesion and its surgical treatment.

- Some people convince themselves that they have a malignant lesion but are reluctant to admit it
- Others have misunderstood the discussion with their primary care doctor and believe that the lesion should be removed. In these circumstances strong reassurance combined with an explanation of the natural history of the lesion may be sufficient
- Some people decide against treatment when they are informed about the technique and risk of scarring

There are some situations in which it may be reasonable to remove a benign lesion:

- Simply because it is very large or unsightly
- It is on a prominent site such as the tip of the nose
- Fleshy moles may catch on clothing
- Skin tags can be unsightly and uncomfortable
- Some lesions, e.g. cysts can become infected and painful

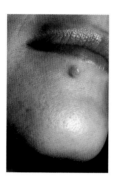

Benign mole on chin

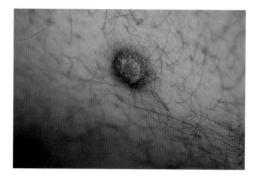

Dermatofibroma with characteristic pigment in a circle around it

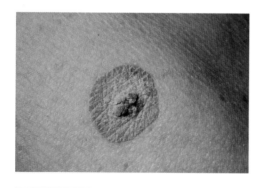

Seborrhoeic keratosis

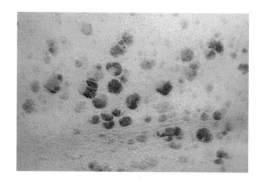

Multiple seborrhoeic keratoses

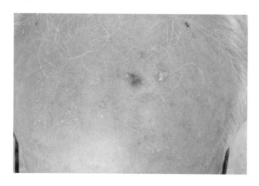

Minor sun damage

No treatment might be best – low-risk lesions

If an elderly and frail individual develops a low-grade premalignant lesion such as a solar keratosis, Bowen's disease or lentigo maligna, it is sometimes the right decision to wait and see – unless it is causing symptoms or problems such as catching on clothing.

The risks of doing nothing

- Each solar keratosis has a 1:1000 chance of malignant change per annum
- Patches of Bowen's disease have 5–20% life-time risk of malignant change
- Lentigo maligna has 10% life-time risk of malignant change
- It is possible for any of the lesions to grow more quickly (see next section)

Healing problems which might occur in elderly people include:

- Slow healing or ulceration of wounds on the lower leg
- Swelling or bruising after use of liquid nitrogen or topical creams

Even when dealing with low-grade malignancy in low-risk sites, there may be an argument to wait and see, particularly in people suffering from other serious illnesses. When dealing with more aggressive lesions it would be unusual not to intervene.

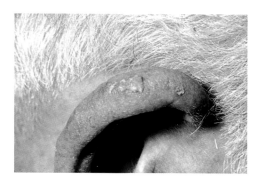

Low-risk solar keratosis

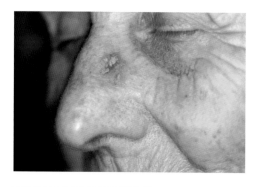

Larger solar keratosis

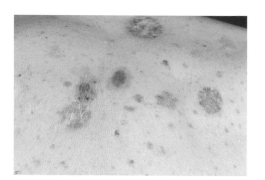

Patches of Bowen's disease

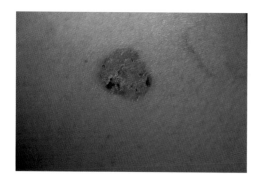

Superficial scaly basal cell carcinoma

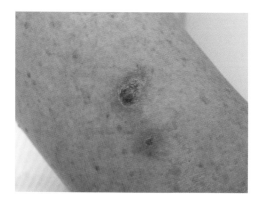

Small nodular basal cell carcinoma (low-risk)

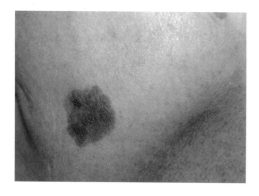

Lentigo maligna

Possible poor outcome from no treatment – benign lesions

The natural history of skin lesions varies enormously. Some benign lesions may reach large proportions while some malignant lesions may be remarkably slow-growing and non-aggressive. The doctor cannot predict exactly what will happen but may be able to give guidance on the likely outcome.

Patients often worry that if they leave a benign lesion to enlarge it will be much more difficult to treat and will leave a much more obvious scar – this is rarely the case, although some lesions do continue to grow.

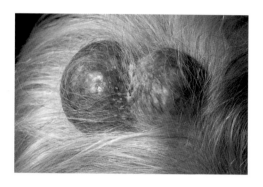

Large scalp cysts

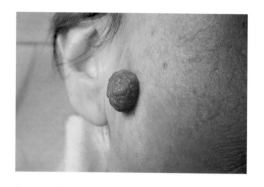

Huge benign mole

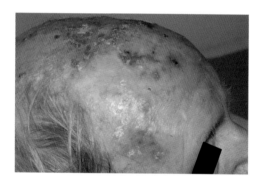

Extensive solar keratosis

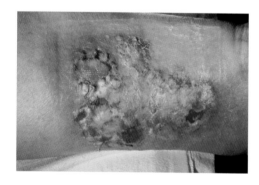

Neglected Bowen's disease

Possible poor outcome from no treatment

Basal cell carcinoma

By definition basal cell carcinomas are malignant tumours. Fortunately they do not spread to internal organs but they can be very destructive on the skin and involve other tissues such as cartilage and bone.

Because they grow slowly and produce few symptoms, it is common for people to neglect them for long periods. Once the diagnosis has been made, it is best to undergo some form of treatment within a few months.

Squamous cell carcinoma

Squamous cell carcinomas are generally more aggressive tumours than basal cell carcinomas. They tend to grow more quickly and invade other tissues, and they can spread to other organs via the lymphatics or blood vessels.

There are very few circumstances in which treatment should not go ahead within a few weeks.

Malignant melanoma

Malignant melanoma is a worrying tumour because its behaviour is so unpredictable. Thick lesions are less likely to be cured than thin ones. For this reason it is important to remove a melanoma as soon as possible and preferably whilst it is still less than 1 mm thick.

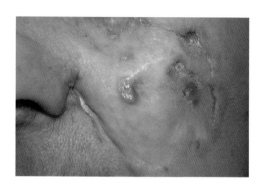

Large infiltrating basal cell carcinoma covering much of the cheek

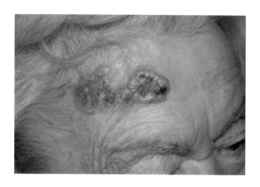

Neglected basal cell carcinoma

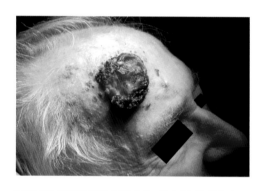

Neglected squamous cell carcinoma

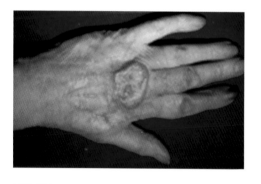

Fast growing squamous cell carcinoma

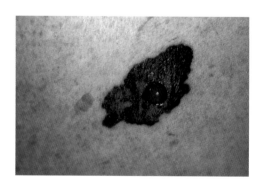

Melanoma with nodule

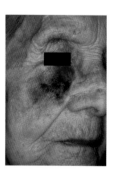

Extensive melanoma

Curettage, cautery, snip, shave, trichloroacetic acid

Curettage

Curettage and cautery are used when the material being removed is softer than the surrounding skin or there is a natural plane to separate the diseased tissue from the normal. It is therefore best for superficial lesions such as:

- Viral warts
- Seborrhoeic warts
- Solar keratosis
- Bowen's disease
- Some forms of skin cancer

It leaves the skin with a graze-like injury, although for skin cancers it has to be a little deeper than a graze. It is usual to cauterize any small blood vessels, and this may give a blackened appearance. Healing is similar to that of a graze and although in some areas it is almost invisible there are some potential minor problems.

Advantages

- Diagnosis can be confirmed histologically
- Usually excellent cosmetic result
- Often single treatment is curative

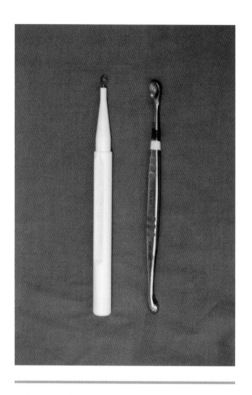

Ring and spoon types of curette

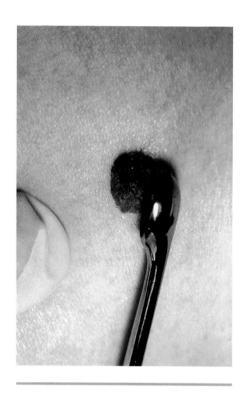

Spoon type curette in action

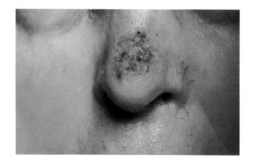

Graze-like appearance
immediately after curettage and
cautery

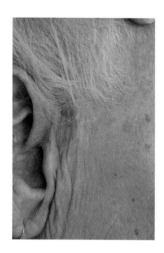

Good healing of a wound

Curettage

Disadvantages

There is always an alternative to curettage so the advantages must be weighed up against the disadvantages:

- Slow healing in areas of friction and on the lower limb
- Altered pigmentation
- A raised or lumpy scar
- Infection of the wound surface
- Bleeding
- A depressed scar

Success rates

There is little published evidence for the cure rates with curettage for benign lesions.

- Most experts agree that it is only about 50–70% effective when treating viral warts but much less so for verrucae on the foot. People with single long-standing warts may have a better chance of success as their immune system has managed to contain the spread of the virus
- It is probably about 95% effective for seborrhoeic keratoses
- If basal cell carcinomas are chosen carefully regarding size, growth pattern and site, it is possible to achieve 90% cure

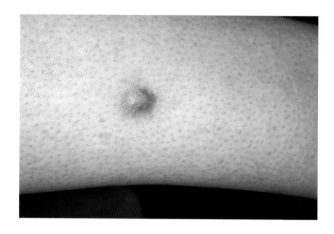

Lumpy scar on lower leg months after curettage and cautery

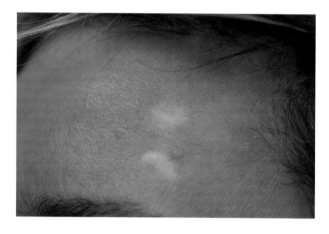

Indented and pale scars months after curettage and cautery

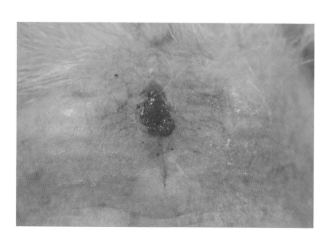

Granulation after curettage and cautery

Electrocautery

Electrocautery and electrodessication are used to destroy small areas of abnormal skin such as tags and prominent blood vessels, and also to cauterize vessels after curettage and shave excision.

At low power this can be done without local anaesthetic. Because it is a destructive method there is always the likelihood of some permanent scar or indentation.

General uses of cautery

- Plane warts
- Small seborrhoeic warts
- Spider naevi and other telangiectasia
- Xanthelasma

Possible side effects

- Indented scar
- Recurrence of lesion

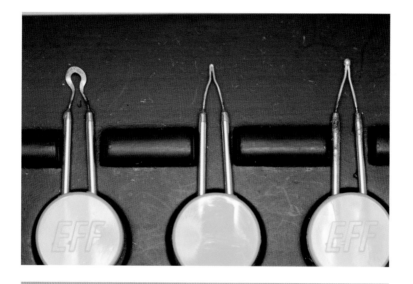

Electrocautery tips

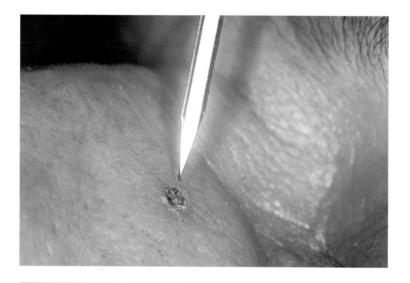

Monopolar hyfrecator tip in action

Snip excision

Lesions on stalks, such as skin tags, are often best treated by snipping the base with sharp scissors. Usually, this does not require anaesthetic. The small amount of bleeding stops with a little pressure. Generally these lesions are not sent for histology.

Large tags and fibroepithelial polyps have a broad base and anaesthetic is used, not only because the snip itself will be more painful but also because cautery may be needed to stop the bleeding.

There are few complications but the following may be a problem:

- Bleeding
- Infection of the base, especially in body folds (e.g. the groin)
- Discomfort if many lesions require treatment
- Slow healing of larger lesions
- Small indented scars

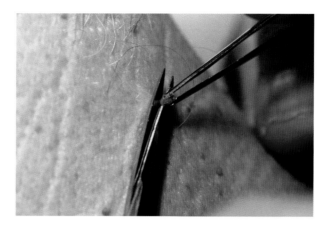

Snipping a skin tag

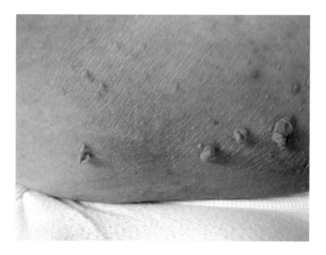

Polyps for snip

Shave excision

Shave excision is one of the simplest procedures to perform. It involves injecting some anaesthetic, shaving the lesion with a blade and finally stopping any bleeding.

For larger lesions a broader blade is used.

This method does not remove the entire lesion, and it therefore allows regrowth in a number of cases. However, for a benign lesion it is often a good treatment.

Benefits

- Simple technique
- 45% of head and neck lesions and 30% of trunk lesions leave no visible scar
- Tissue is available for analysis

Problems (approximate figures)

- 25% of pigmented lesions have residual pigment
- Rarely, pigment appears in a previously non-pigmented mole
- Terminal hairs remain in 20%
- Occasional doughnut-shaped scar
- Rarely, infection
- Rarely, regrowth of the lesion

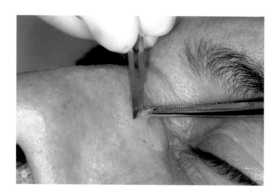

Shave excision of a papular lesion on nose

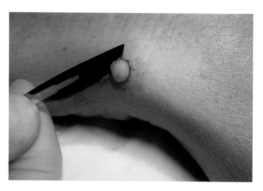

Shave excision of a broader-based lesion

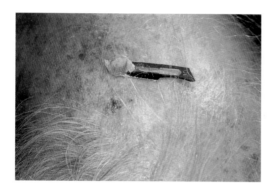

Diagnostic shave biopsy

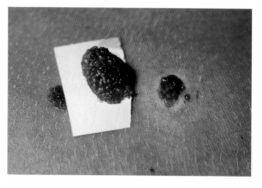

Shave excision of a large warty naevus

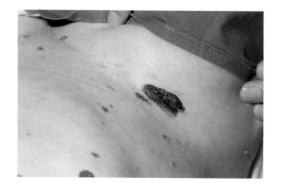

Seborrhoeic keratosis

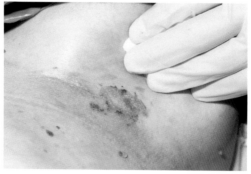

Seborrhoeic keratosis after shave excision

Shave excision of raised moles

Pathologically benign raised moles may be a cosmetic problem on the face and can catch on clothing or jewellery at other sites. In these situations there is a high rate of satisfaction from treatment but as with all other techniques there are some potential problems:

- Occasionally the scar becomes raised or slightly lumpy
- The flat scar may become much darker than before
- If it ever becomes necessary to operate again on a regrowing mole it can be difficult to interpret the pathology
- On the face there is sometimes a slightly sunken appearance

Biopsy of tumours

Shave biopsy of a tumour produces a good specimen for analysis. It does not usually attempt to care the tumour unless a deeper saucerisation is performed. In this case a more obvious scar can be expected.

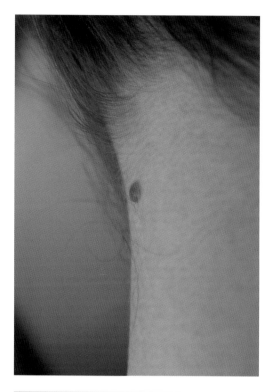

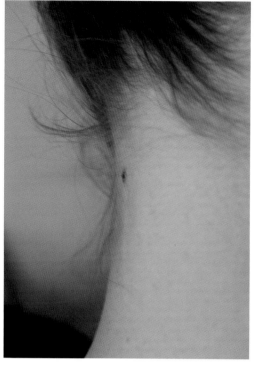

Papular lesion on the neck

Papular lesion on the neck after shave and cautery

Trichloroacetic acid

Acids can be used to destroy superficial lesions. Trichloroacetic acid is used at strengths from 10% to 90%. Soon after the acid comes into contact with the skin it becomes inactivated, but depending on the strength and the number of applications, it can produce significant superficial destruction.

Facial peels

It is used in weak solutions for facial peels in rejuvenation treatments. It can be applied more locally to deal with age spots and small keratoses.

Xanthelasma

Many doctors use trichloroacetic acid to treat the fatty deposits which may form around the eyes known as xanthelasma. There is a marked difference between the way individuals will react, and some will get considerable swelling (and usually very good clearance) whereas others react to a lesser degree. Occasionally scarring occurs. Also these lesions tend to recur so that treatment at intervals of a few year may be necessary. Surgical excision has also been used but it they recur the amount of available skin for further excision is limited.

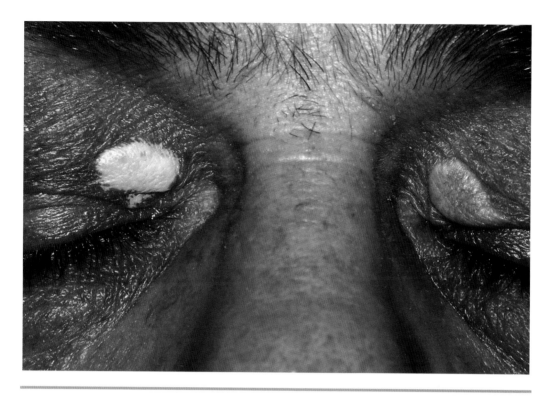

Frosting on a xanthelasma of the right eye immediately after application of trichloroacetic acid

Cryosurgery

Introduction

Cryosurgery is used in dermatology more frequently than any other physical treatment. It is readily available and no preparation of the skin is required. Over the last 20 years liquid nitrogen has become the most popular freezing medium and it can be delivered either on a cotton swab or through a spray nozzle. It is extremely cold, at −196°C.

Alternatives to cryosurgery

Other freezing treatments include over-the-counter 'Wartner', which contains dimethyl ether and propane. The coldest temperature it reaches is −57°C, so the temperatures deeper in the tissues are often not sufficient. 'Histofreeze' contains the same ingredients.

Use of liquid nitrogen

- Short treatment times are used to treat minor sun damage, warts and some cosmetically troublesome blemishes
- Longer treatment times are needed to treat more resistant lesions such as certain skin cancers
- It must be remembered that cryosurgery is a destructive tool and can produce surprising effects after relatively non-aggressive treatment schedules
- Many of the changes that occur after freezing tissue are inflammatory and are important in the success of the treatment. In other words, absence of 'side effects' may result in absence of any benefit
- Some of the unwanted effects are specific to the site, pathology and size of the lesion

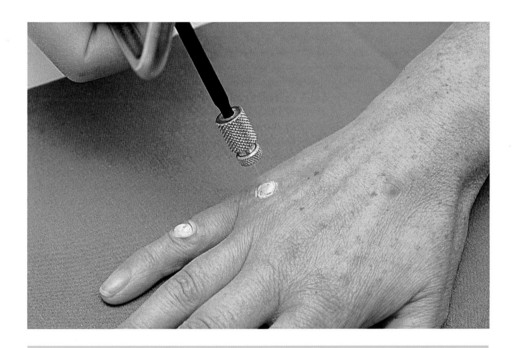

Ice ball appearing on the skin with liquid nitrogen

Benefits

Cryosurgery can be performed in the primary care setting or in the hospital setting as an outpatient procedure. It is quick and generally leaves good cosmetic results. For harmless skin lesions it can be repeated if necessary.

Seborrhoeic keratosis

Despite widespread use there are few data available on the success rate. For thin lesions it is nearly always successful. Very thick keratoses, on the other hand, may be quite resistant.

Warts and verrucae

There is a long running debate about the value of liquid nitrogen. Most studies and a major review of all past studies conclude that:

- At its best it is as good as wart paints on the hand
- It is generally quite effective for facial warts
- It is generally poor for verrucae on the feet

Chondrodermatitis

These painful nodules on the ear respond in around 50% of cases, but relapse is also seen. It is sometimes worth trying cryotherapy initially and going on to other treatments if it recurs. Fairly long treatment times are needed. It is also important to take measures after treatment to relieve pressure on the ear so as to avoid recurrence.

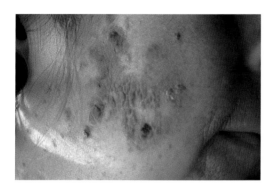

Large seborrhoeic keratoses on the
cheek

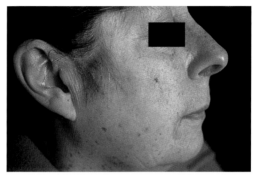

Cheek 6 weeks after cryosurgery

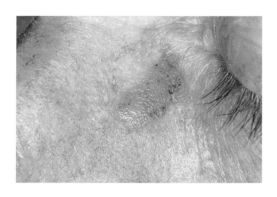

Seborrhoeic keratosis by the eye

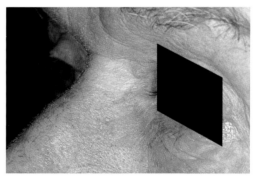

Same eye area 3 months after
cryosurgery

Pigmented lesions

If there is any doubt about the diagnosis of a pigmented lesion it is unwise to use cryosurgery because it may mask the progress of a malignant lesion at a later date. It is rarely used on moles. Some pigmented lesions do respond to this treatment:

- Simple lentigo
- Solar lentigo
- Some pigmentations on the lips

Solar keratosis

Solar keratosis is one of the lesions most frequently seen by dermatologists and there are many ways to deal with them. The method depends to some extent on the thickness of the lesion and the extent of the sun damage.

- Early fairly flat, scaly lesions often respond well to cryosurgery
- Small raised lesions may respond
- Keratosis on the lip can be treated in this way
- Thicker lesions do not respond well and demand other treatments
- Overall, using a double freeze–thaw cycle cryosurgery has been found to give a complete response in 75% of solar keratoses after a single treatment when assessed at 3 months. Even with thick lesions it was 69%

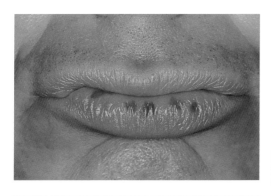
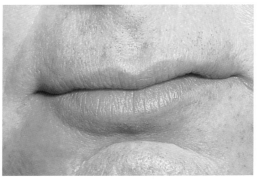

Pigmented lesions on the lips

Area 3 months after treatment

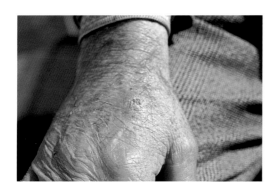
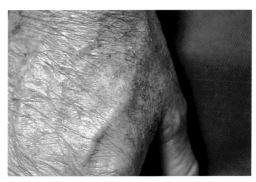

Solar keratosis

Area 6 weeks after treatment

Bowen's disease

There are many ways to treat Bowen's disease, and informed choice is important. Cryosurgery has the advantage that it can be performed immediately, in the consulting room. Bowen's disease often occurs on the lower leg and healing can be slow.

In one study using liquid nitrogen with two freeze–thaw cycles of 20 seconds each for 82 lesions on the lower leg, there were recurrences in five patients (6%) after a 1-year follow-up. No anaesthesia was required, and there were no treatment-related failures of healing.

Another study reported 100% clearance in 20 patients after between one and three treatments with liquid nitrogen using one freeze–thaw cycle of 20 seconds on each occasion (50% success after a single treatment). There were two recurrences (10%) in the 1-year follow-up period.

Cryotherapy therefore appears to have a good success rate (with recurrences in less than 10% at 12 months), but healing may be slow for broad lesions, and discomfort may limit treatment of multiple lesions.

Skin cancer

Generally it is only low-grade skin cancers that are treated with cryosurgery. The doses involved are greater than for warts and keratoses. The side effects are therefore greater, and wounds can be inflamed and discharge for 2–3 weeks before scabbing over. However the cosmetic results are often good, and it is rare to get distortion.

For superficial basal cell carcinoma the success rate is over 95% and for small low-risk nodular tumours it is over 90%.

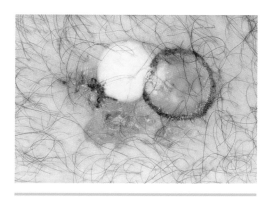

Bowen's disease treated in overlapping circles

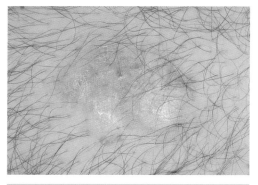

Area of treatment 3 months later

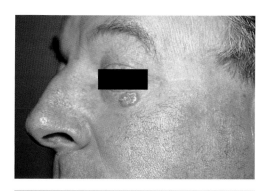

Basal cell cancer on lower eyelid

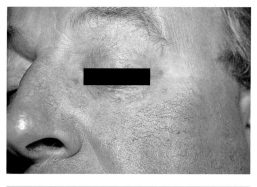

Area 3 months after treatment

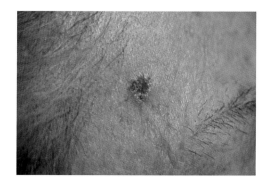

Basal cell carcinoma on the temple

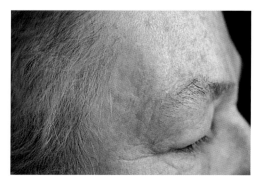

Area of treatment 18 weeks later

Side effects and complications

Immediate effects

- Pain
- Swelling
- Blister formation

Pain

Cryosurgery is an uncomfortable procedure and it is generally not recommended for children under the age of 7–10 years, depending on how brave they are.

- Everyone feels some discomfort
- Even the shortest freezes give a perceptible 'hot' or 'burning' sensation and bigger doses can be quite painful
- The pain may settle quickly only to be replaced by further discomfort during the thaw phase – sometimes lasting for many minutes
- Certain areas are more painful – the fingers, ears, lips, temples and scalp
- Even though pain as described above is usually transient, a throbbing sensation may persist for 1–2 hours

Swelling (oedema)

Some swelling is seen with every patient, and it is an expected outcome of the acute inflammation and 'leaky' capillaries. The amount of swelling relates to the length and depth of the treatment.

- Generally, short freezes for cosmetic blemishes will not lead to much swelling
- After large doses for skin cancers the area will always become swollen and often blister
- Unexpected oedema, sometimes with blood-stained blistering, occasionally occurs, even after short freeze schedules
- The severest oedema is typically seen in lax skin sites – e.g. the eyelids, lips and genital skin. Such blisters are often painless

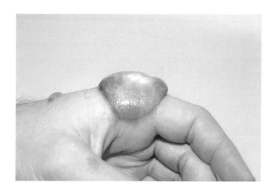

Blood-filled blister after wart treatment

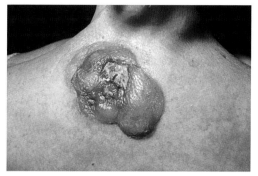

Large blister on the back

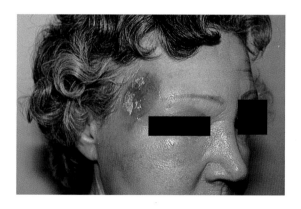

Swelling may cause the eye to close

Side effects and complications

Delayed effects

- Vascular necrosis
- Infection
- Bleeding
- Granulation tissue

Note that:

- occasionally bleeding occurs soon after thawing and is related to cracks which appear in the ice ball during freezing
- within 4–7 days of aggressive cryosurgery it is not uncommon for the treated field to become blue or purple, with subsequent necrosis and sloughing of the dead tissue
- if cryosurgery is preceded by biopsy or curettage (e.g. to debulk a tumour) then bleeding is more common as it thaws
- although discharge and yellow discoloration is common this is usually not due to infection. However, if pain increases after a few days then infection should be suspected

The rarest and most dramatic form of haemorrhage can be delayed by up to 14 days after treatment. It may be caused by delayed necrosis of a tumour that had already invaded blood vessels. Bleeding of this type may be profuse. It requires immediate pressure to minimize blood loss, and early medical attention.

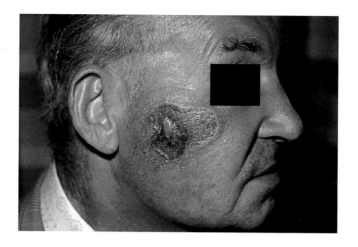

Vascular necrosis 6 days after aggressive
cryosurgery

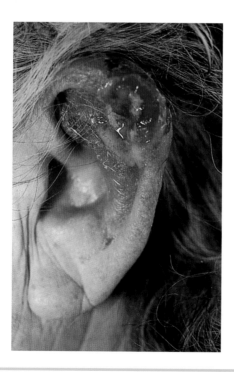

Necrosis of tissue at 1 week after cryosurgery
can give the impression of infection

Side effects and complications

Prolonged effects

Some prolonged effects are usually temporary:

- Increased pigmentation
- Milia (tiny white cysts)
- Hypertrophic scars
- Numbness at the site of treatment

Pigment changes are unpredictable but it is risky to use cryosurgery on people with dark skins because depigmentation may be permanent. In people of all skin types, prolonged pale patches are common, and initially there may be a halo of darker skin, which highlights it even more.

Other prolonged effects are usually permanent:

- Decreased pigmentation
- Loss of hair follicles
- Notching of eyelids, cartilage or lips after large doses. If a skin cancer has already invaded tissues they will inevitably necrose after cryosurgery. The nail matrix and tendon can be damaged around the nail folds
- Sensory impairment

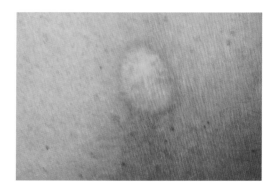

Increased pigment at the edge of a
pale scar following cryosurgery

Hypertrophic scar on the leg

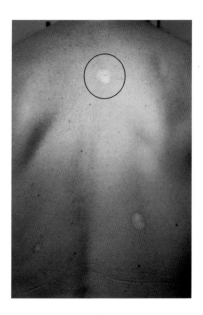

Permanent loss of pigment
(area circled on upper back)

Side effects and complications

Prolonged effects

Aggressive treatments, usually for skin cancer, may damage underlying structures. Scars are usually flat but may be slightly indented, thinned or thickened.

Some degree of paraesthesia is common after freezing. If a nerve trunk underlying a treated skin lesion is inadvertently damaged, complete recovery of distal sensory or motor function can be expected.

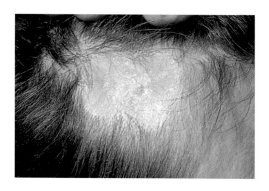

Scarring and hair loss on the scalp

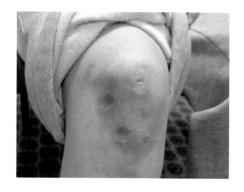

Sunken scars at the site of wart treatment

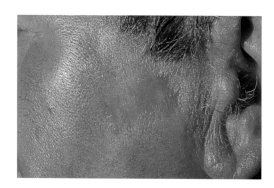

Loss of tissue following skin cancer treatment

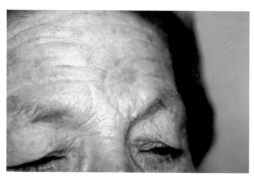

Severe atrophic scar after skin cancer treatment

Side effects and complications

Prolonged effects in cartilage

Cartilage is fairly resistant to the damaging effects of cryosurgery. However, if the tumour has invaded cartilage prior to treatment then there will be inevitable loss of tissue after treatment.

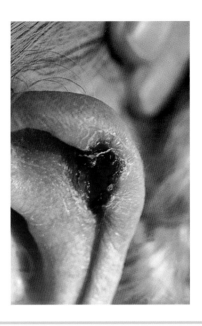

Eroding basal cell carcinoma
affecting the helix

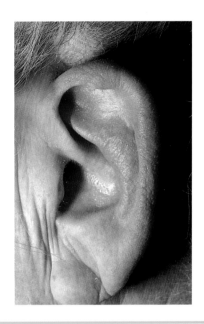

Excellent resolution with minimal
cartilage loss

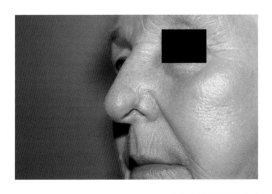

Notching of the alar rim after skin
cancer treatment

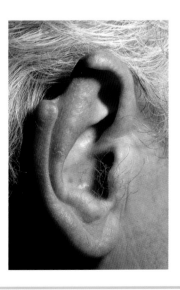

Severe cartilage loss after skin cancer
treatment

Radiotherapy

Introduction

Ionizing radiation has been used to treat skin cancers for more than 100 years. Despite advances in surgical and other treatment modalities, radiotherapy still has an important role in the management of skin tumours.

The radiation source is either a high-energy electron beam (particulate) or superficial X-rays (photons). The electron beam causes less damage to underlying cartilage and bone but is more complex to deliver.

Low-dose radiation may trigger development of basal cell carcinoma and squamous cell carcinoma, as historically seen following treatment for ringworm of the scalp and ankylosing spondylitis. However, higher doses of radiation can effectively cure these and other skin tumours.

Radiotherapy can be effective in treating many skin cancers:

• Basal cell carcinoma
• Squamous cell carcinoma and keratoacanthoma
• Lentigo maligna
• Merkel cell tumour
• Malignant melanoma (palliative therapy)
• Lymphoma

Some tumours are not suitable for radiotherapy:

• Sweat gland and adnexal tumours
• Atypical fibroxanthoma
• Dermatofibrosarcoma protuberans

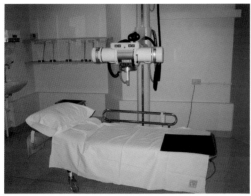

Superficial radiotherapy

Treatment tube in place over lesion

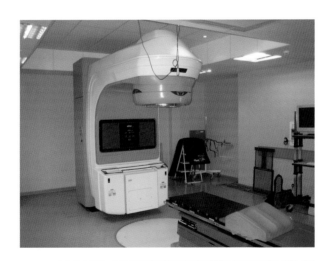

Linear accelerator

Advantages

- Painless and does not need anaesthetic
- Useful for patients unsuitable for surgery
- Less destructive than surgery at some sites (e.g. the lip, the ear)
- May be useful to treat incompletely excised or recurrent tumours

Disadvantages

- No margin control
- Requires tertiary referral and multiple visits
- Cannot be repeated if treatment fails
- Less suitable in those under 60 years of age because of poor long-term cosmetic results
- Long-term risk of inducing secondary malignancy in the treatment field

Typical treatment regimes			
SIZE OF TUMOUR	DOSE OF RADIATION	NUMBER OF FRACTIONS (I.E. NUMBER OF VISITS)	DURATION OF COURSE
Up to 2.5 cm	27 Gy	3	2 weeks
OR	35 Gy	5	1 week
Up to 4.5 cm	45 Gy	10	2 weeks
Greater than 4.5 cm	50 Gy	15	3 weeks

Schedules may vary with local protocols. Occasionally a single fraction may be prescribed to treat a very small tumour. In general, the greater the number of fractions, the better the long-term cosmetic result. Different regimes apply for treatment of recurrent, nodal or metastatic disease.

Higher-energy radiotherapy (140 kV instead of 100 kV) is used to treat thicker skin cancers, and the radiation penetrates more deeply.

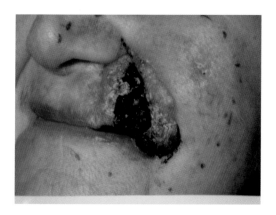

Huge skin cancer on the lip

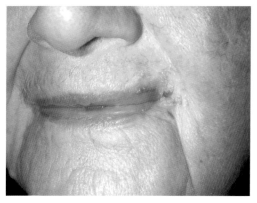

Area after successful radiotherapy

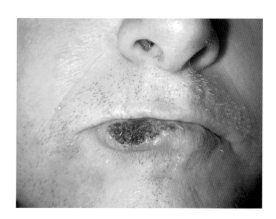

Carcinoma on the lip

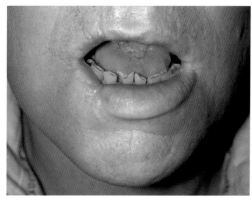

Area after radiotherapy

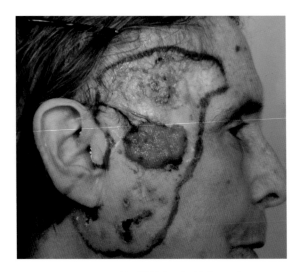

Huge basal cell carcinoma

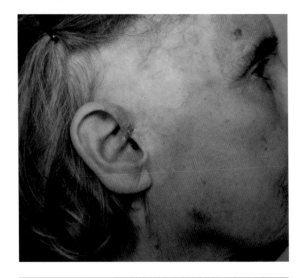

Area after radiotherapy

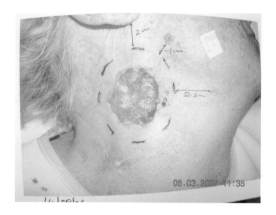

Large tumour before radiotherapy

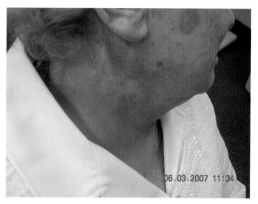

Months after treatment

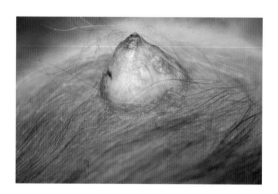

Tumour on scalp

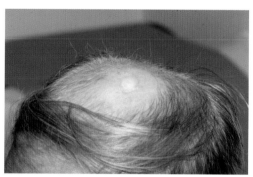

Following treatment

Side effects

Early effects (first 2 weeks)

- Erythema
- Oozing and occasional ulceration
- Crusting

Intermediate effects

- Hypopigmentation and possible later hyperpigmentation
- Telangiectasia
- Atrophy
- Loss of hair

Late effects

- Radionecrosis (particularly below the neck, over joints or bones and at areas of friction); radionecrosis may appear as a non-healing ulcerated area within the treatment scar, and can be mistaken for recurrent tumour and biopsy may be required to differentiate
- Cataract if treatment is near the eye
- Dry eye if the lachrymal apparatus is within the treatment area
- Recurrence of tumour (5 year cure rates around 90%)
- Rarely, development of a new primary tumour in the treatment field may be required to distinguish the two

Patients undergoing superficial radiotherapy for skin cancer do not experience pain or systemic effects (e.g. sickness, malaise) as they may do with treatment of internal cancers.

Most treatment sites are healed within 6 weeks of the start of radiotherapy.

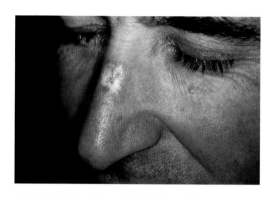

Pale old radiotherapy scar

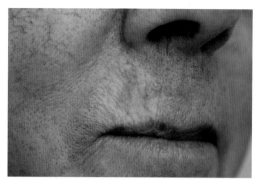

Discoloured old scar

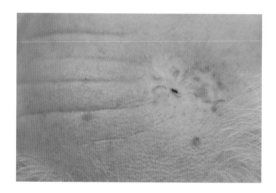

Sunken scar with small vessels
prominent

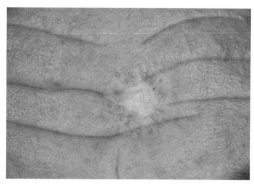

Pale, mottled scar

Biopsies and excisions

Biopsies and small excisions

Some individuals heal better than others but the quality of the final scar is unpredictable. Body site is important – areas such as the chest are more likely to produce hypertrophic scars, and the lower legs heal much more slowly than the upper body.

Other complications which can lead to a poor scar are:

- Bleeding – haematoma formation
- Allergic reactions
- Infection
- Wound separation – dehiscence
- Suturing complications
- Hypertrophic scars
- Stretched scars
- Pigmentary changes
- Unexplained odd healing
- Previous radiotherapy at the site

- It is impossible to predict the quality of a scar, even after small procedures
- Sometimes diagnostic biopsies lead to unsightly, hypertrophic scars

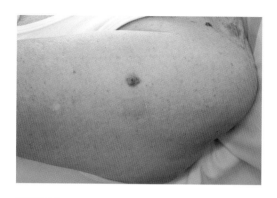

Small lesion before removal

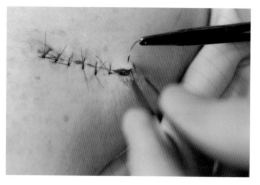

Suturing nearly complete

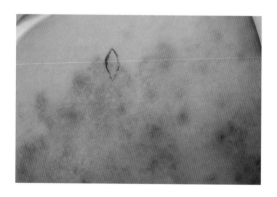

Rash before biopsy

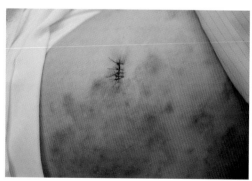

Biopsy complete

Diagnostic biopsy, punch biopsy and small excisions

The principles are the same for all procedures in which the full thickness of the skin is removed. The overall impact will be much less with small procedures but it is important to be aware that although good results are the norm it is possible to have complications from minimal surgical intervention.

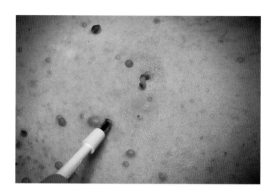

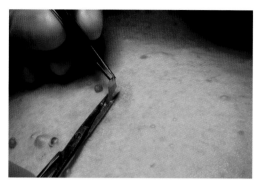

Small punch biopsy removing a core of skin

Removing the specimen

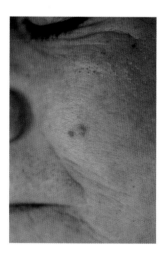

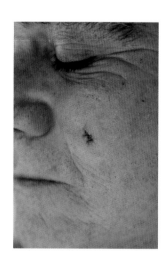

Small lesion before biopsy

Immediately after biopsy

Diagnostic biopsy, punch biopsy and small excisions

If a skin lesion is being removed for cosmetic reasons it is very important to be aware of the possible outcomes. Sometimes the final scar is worse than the original problem.

Invisible mending is not possible after skin surgery – however, the majority of scars settle very well. Whether a patient is happy with the results depends on his or her expectation. It is easy to get the impression, from glossy magazines, that near-invisible surgery should be expected. The pictures here show some good results but small scars are still visible.

At other times the scar looks worse than the original for months before eventually settling down. It can take up to 18 months for the fully mature scar to develop – after that there is unlikely to be a significant change in appearance or texture.

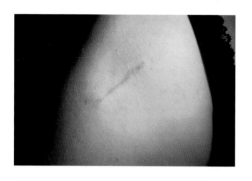

Fair result on the shoulder

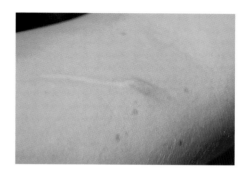

Good scar but one end has been slower to heal

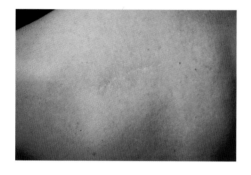

Good result on the back

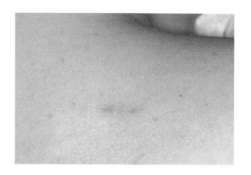

Final result

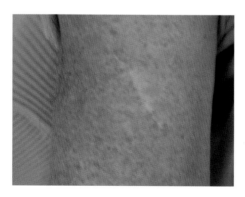

Good scar after small excision

Diagnostic biopsy, punch biopsy and small excisions

Complications

It is perhaps surprising how many problems there can be with small biopsies and excisions. Wound infections, wound dehiscence and hypertrophic scars are not infrequent. It makes the decision to take a biopsy more difficult, especially if the only suitable site is in a cosmetically important area. An example would be a rash on the cheeks. If the rash clears completely at a later stage it is possible that the only visible mark left will be the biopsy scar – and if it is a slightly raised or spread scar the disappointment will be even greater.

When to take the stitches out?

If stitches are left in for too long there will be permanent stitch marks. If they are taken out too soon there is the possibility of the wound bursting open. One way to overcome this is to insert buried, self-dissolving sutures first. Often this is the correct approach but in thin skin it may be impossible, or they may stick out through the scar for weeks or months.

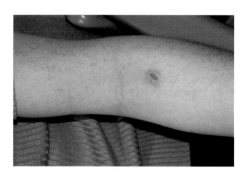

Infection of a small wound on the leg

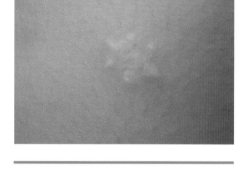

Prominent stitch marks in a 10-year-old patient

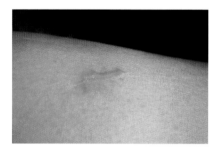

Lumpy scar on the arm post-biopsy

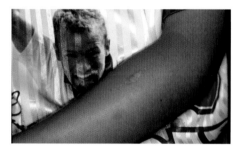

Poor scar following mole removal

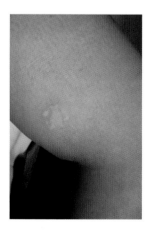

Spread scar on the leg

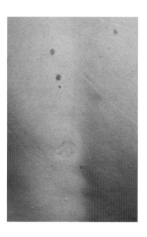

Stretched scar on the back

Larger excisions

Some individuals heal better than others but the quality of the final scar is unpredictable. Some variables can be assessed to give a relative risk of outcome. Elderly people and those on long-term corticosteroids may have thinner skin. Body site is also important – areas such as the chest are more likely to produce hypertrophic scars, and the lower legs heal much more slowly than the upper body.

Other complications which can lead to a poor scar are shown on the page opposite.

- It is impossible to predict the quality of a scar, even after small procedures
- Healing is an unpredictable event
- Sometimes long scars fade to become almost imperceptible while some small scars persist as visible blemishes

Possible complications

Bleeding and haematoma	May occur within hours or be delayed
Infection	Seen most with ulcerated lesions and on the lower limb
Wound separation (dehiscence)	May occur with infection or if the wound is under tension
Suturing complications	Deeper stitches may 'spit' or work their way out. Stitch marks are often seen when stitches are left in for more than 1 week
Hypertrophic scars and keloid	Unpredictable unless there is a previous history of the same
Stretched and sunken scars	Quite common on the back or if the wound is under tension
Pigmentary change	More common in skin types 3–6
Redness and telangiectasia	May take long time to settle
Distortion and 'dog-ears'	More commonly seen in larger excisions
Allergic reactions	Very rare with anaesthetic; reactions to dressings are uncommon
Unexplained poor healing	Rare and unpredictable

Fresh operation site

Some people do not want to see the freshly sutured wound before a dressing is applied. For those who are going to change their own dressing it can be helpful to see it so there is no misunderstanding about the expectation of its appearance.

A few individuals like to watch the actual operation but it is not for the faint-hearted.

The wound often looks swollen because of infiltration of local anaesthetic. It may be pale or mottled because adrenaline constricts blood vessels. There may be a little oozing of blood.

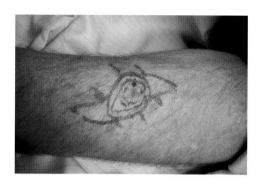

Asymmetric excision – called the 'lazy S'

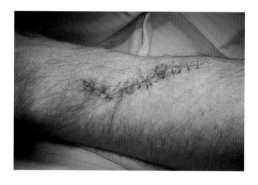

The wound after 24 hours

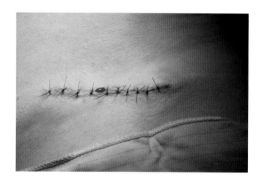

A freshly sutured wound

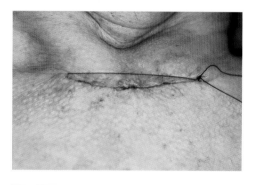

Subcuticular suture in a fresh wound

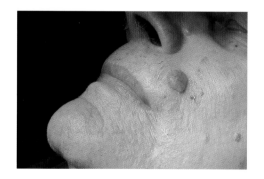

A lesion on the lip

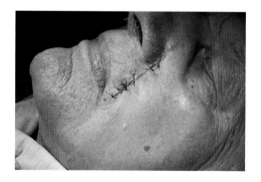

Area immediately after closure

Larger excisions with primary closure

Good results

The pictures on the right show several examples of larger excisions at different sites. In all cases it has been possible to bring the wound edges together (or almost so) without undue tension producing a satisfactory closure.

The direction of closure depends on the shape of the lesion to be removed, the natural folds in the skin and the relaxed skin tension lines. On the forehead it is often best to close in a vertical line, rather than horizontally along the forehead creases. It can be described as choosing a line as in a sundial, so that in the middle of the forehead the closure will be vertical but further out towards the temple the line will be increasingly at an angle.

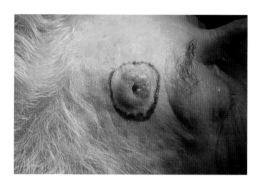

Large tumour above the outer
aspect of the eyebrow

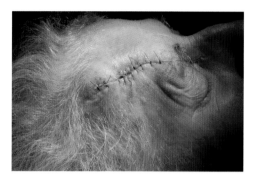

Wound closed in an almost
vertical direction

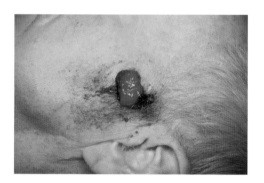

Large lesion in front of the left ear

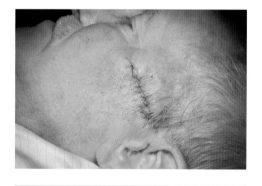

Wound closed horizontally

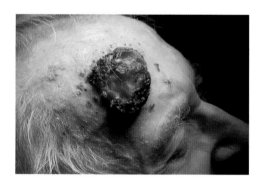

Huge lesion on the forehead

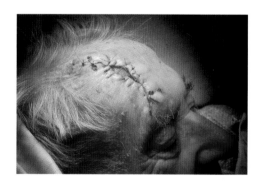

It is not always possible to get
primary closure

Larger excisions with primary closure

Good results

The pictures on the right show several examples of larger excisions at different sites. In all cases it has been possible to bring the wound edges together without undue tension producing a satisfactory closure.

Some sites are more prone to hypertrophic scars but as seen in the picture opposite the chest can heal extremely well in some cases.

Deeper excisions

Sometimes it is necessary to remove all the fat underlying a skin lesion e.g. when removing a malignant melanoma. This more often leads to a slightly indented scar and it can be quite noticeable on the upper arm and leg.

When removing malignant lesions there is thought to be an advantage if the skin can be closed primarily because it is less disruptive to the lymph vessels and the normal anatomy. If flaps are used there is the possibility of moving some remaining malignant cells to a new position in relation to the scar as well as damaging more lymph vessels – and they have an important function for the immune system. Grafts are acceptable as they do not further alter the local tissues.

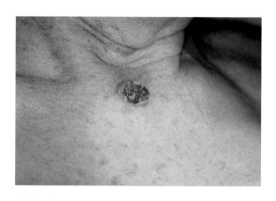

Skin cancer on the chest

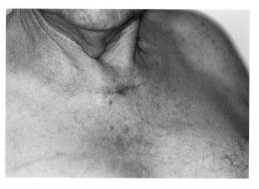

Good healing of the wound

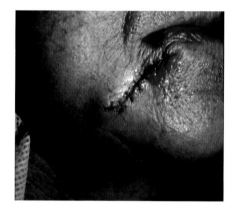

Lesion removed from the chin

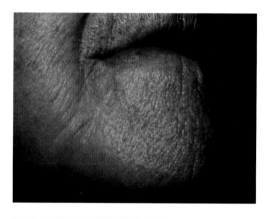

Good healing several months later

5

Larger excisions with good results

The majority of scars heal well, and at the time of suture removal the scar already looks healthy.

Stitches are left in for varying times, ranging from a few days to 3 weeks, depending on body site and the type of closure used. The head and neck always heal more quickly because of the excellent blood supply.

General advice to encourage good healing

- Go home and rest
- Avoid over-exertion and bending down
- Use extra pillows after facial surgery and elevate the leg after lower limb surgery
- Do not drink alcohol or smoke for 48 hours
- Use paracetamol rather than aspirin for pain relief
- If bleeding occurs apply firm pressure for 20 minutes using a clean handkerchief over the dressing
- Avoid going out in very cold weather

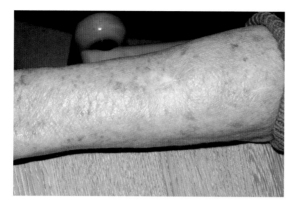

Good mature scar on forearm

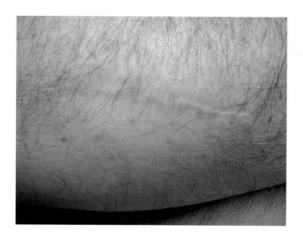

Fair result for large scar on limb

Good and minimally suboptimal results

Some areas heal less well than others, so that a result considered to be good when seen on the back might be regarded as suboptimal if the same scar were seen on the face.

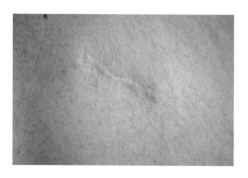

A 4 cm scar on the back – a good result

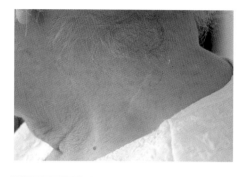

A good mature scar on the neck

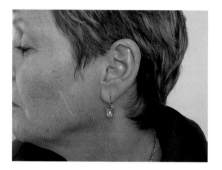

A good mature scar on the cheek

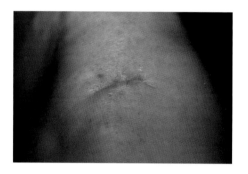

A slightly raised scar, but a fair result on the shoulder

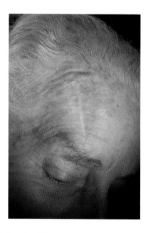

A long mature scar on the forehead

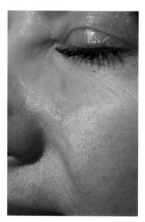

A reasonable scar after mole removal

Bleeding, bruising and haematoma

Some bleeding is an inevitable part of a surgical procedure but it can also be a problem. Unexpected bleeding may occur for a number of reasons, discussed below.

Diseases that make bleeding more likely

These include inherited diseases such as haemophilia, and conditions that lead to a low platelet count or reduced platelet function e.g. chronic lymphatic leukaemia.

Drugs that make bleeding more likely

The best-known drug that promotes bleeding is warfarin, and a large number of people now take it. It is important to have a blood test (International Normalized Ratio, INR), usually within 48 hours before surgery, to make sure the blood is not too thin and likely to create bleeding problems. The safe level for the blood test depends to some extent on the nature of the skin surgery, but generally the INR should be lower for bigger operations. For bigger operations most surgeons would prefer the INR to be less than 3.5. Warfarin does not seem to affect bleeding during the operation but makes postoperative bleeding more likely. The likelihood of postoperative bleeding is increased but cannot be predicted by the actual level so long as it is in the therapeutic range.

It is usually safe to continue aspirin but if bleeding is likely to be a significant problem it is best to stop it 14 days before surgery. For clopidogrel the time is 7 days. These drugs should only be stopped in agreement with your general practitioner because there are risks associated with stopping them.

Early postoperative bleeding

Bleeding from the wound before leaving the hospital or in the first 24 hours can be due to the effects of the adrenalin used in the local anaesthetic wearing off. Often the bleeding vessel is in the area of undermining or in muscle. The outer dressing should be removed and firm pressure applied for 15 minutes. If the bleeding does not stop then return to hospital is recommended.

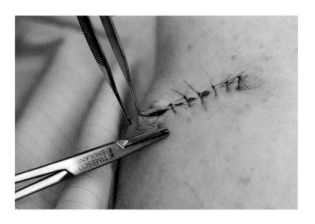

Fresh bleeding at the excision site

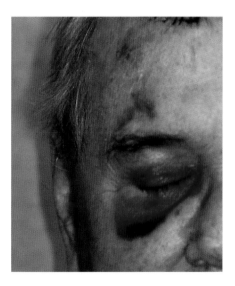

Bruising moved by gravity

Bleeding, bruising and haematoma

Late postoperative bleeding and haematoma

Bruising or a haematoma may form several days later. Late bruising is occasionally due to early postoperative bleeding which has entered a tissue plane and gravitated to a distant site.

Haematomas can be uncomfortable. If they are seen at an early stage it is possible to remove blood through a large-bore needle or by removing one stitch and inserting a small curette. Older haematomas become quite firm and disappear over several months.

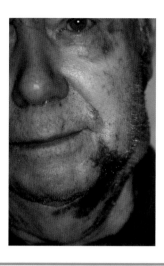

Haematoma and bruising

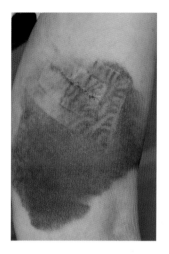

Haematoma on a limb

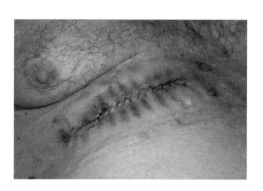

Swelling and bruising; the patient
was on warfarin

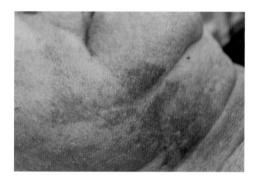

Bruising 1 week after an operation
on the nose

Wound infection

Mild wound infection

A mild wound infection can be difficult to detect because even a healthy wound may have some redness and swelling around it and be slightly tender to touch. Some inflammation may be seen around the sutures. A true infection usually becomes apparent around 4 days postoperatively. There is increasing redness and pain at the time when one would expect decreasing pain. There may be pustules.

Mild infection may clear spontaneously, especially once sutures are removed. However, if pain is experienced it is often necessary to give antibiotics by mouth.

Operations on broken skin are more likely to become infected, as are those performed on skin below the knee, where the incidence is over 5%.

Wet wounds

People have different views about the wisdom of allowing the wound to get wet in the first 48 hours after surgery. A large study did not show any difference in rates of infection between patients who bathed their wounds and those who did not.

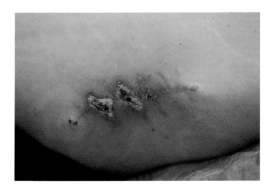

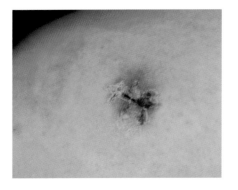

The wound is red but not infected

Redness around the wound, and a pustule

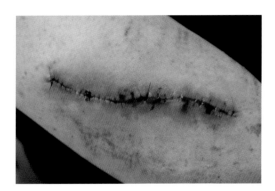

A mild wound infection, which may require antibiotics

Wound infection

Severe wound infection

More aggressive bacteria can produce severe pain and wound break-down. Spreading redness and swelling denote cellulitis, and this must be treated with antibiotics.

Infections impair wound healing and the sutures should be left in for a few days longer.

Regarding viruses, it is important to know that herpes simplex and herpes zoster may reactivate in areas of trauma, including surgical sites. In addition, herpes simplex (the cold sore virus) can be transmitted from the patient's own body or from that of a health-care professional.

Wound infections are more likely on the extremities.

Antibiotics

If antibiotics are required, it is important to:

- Use the right agent – infection is usually due to *Staphylococcus aureus*, and flucloxacillin or clarithromycin are best
- Swab the wound but start antibiotics without waiting for the result
- Use antibiotics for long enough (7–10 days' treatment is often needed)
- Use adequate doses (e.g. 500 mg four times a day in the case of flucloxacillin)
- Remember that infection is much more likely after surgery to ulcerated lesions, after prolonged surgical procedures and after surgery near the nose or on the lower leg

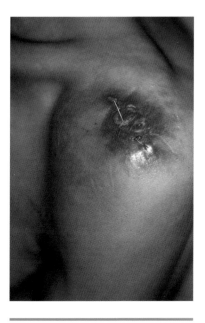

A severe infection

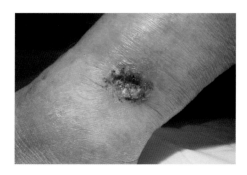

A severe infection with
breakdown

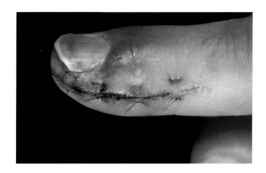

Herpes simplex infection in a
wound

Wound separation (dehiscence)

Wounds gain strength slowly. Often there will be buried stitches, which maintain some strength for several weeks. Several factors can make a wound more likely to break down:

- Haematoma
- Wound infection
- Wound at a site of friction
- Wound under great tension
- Premature removal of sutures
- Smoking habits
- Various underlying medical conditions
- Bending, lifting, etc.
- Shaving – men may shave off the knot of a suture placed on the face; men should avoid shaving the affected area

In the early days after surgery the wound is weak and easily damaged. At day 6, the breaking strength is only about 10% of normal. The wound breaking strength does not reach 45% of normal until day 70; it reaches 50% of normal at day 120. It never reaches more than 80%. With this in mind, it is important to avoid large physical stresses in the first few weeks after surgery.

A wound that has dehisced can sometimes be resutured if the dehiscence happens in the first 24 hours. If the dehiscence is due to haematoma or infection it should be left to heal by secondary intention.

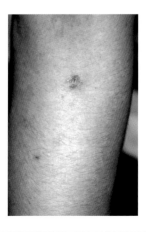

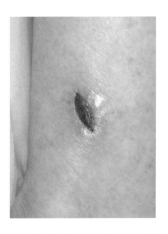

Dehiscence of a wound on the arm

Dehisced wound

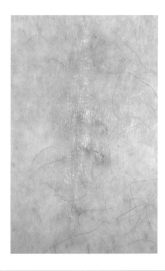

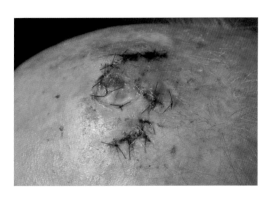

Dehisced wound on scalp

Retained suture material

Suturing complications

Suture tracks

The most common causes of suture tracks are listed below.

- Leaving the stitches in too long. Removing sutures by 7 days generally prevents the marks whereas if sutures are left in for 14 days they are frequent. The explanation is that the epidermis grows into the track; this is most obvious in skin with plentiful adnexal structures. If it has not been possible to place deep sutures the surface ones need to stay in for longer and stitch marks become inevitable
- Tension in the wound. This is also important and can occur when the tissues are advanced a long way or simply as a result of tying the stitches too tight
- Oedema developing after surgery. This may render stitches tight when they had apparently been satisfactory at the time of surgery. Stitches which tear the tissue will inevitably leave extra scarring behind

A stitch mark is less of a problem than a dehisced wound. The use of buried sutures, which support the wound, allow the top stitches to be taken out sooner. However it is not possible to use deep sutures at all sites and especially so when the skin is very thin.

Extrusion of buried sutures ('spitting')

Extrusion of sutures is quite common yet it is not clear why it happens. Every effort is made not to tie the buried suture too high in the dermis and to place the knot at the bottom. Extrusion can be seen as early as 2 weeks or as late as 8 weeks after surgery. A crust followed by an erosion appears, and after a while the top of the suture material can be seen. It is usually possible to cut the suture out without any untoward effect. The spitting stitch sometimes looks like a pustule. Patients often think that this complication, which occurs in the middle of the scar, represents recurrence of the tumour.

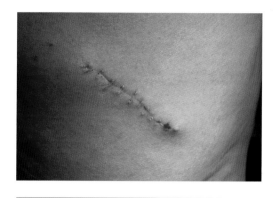

Suture marks just after removal

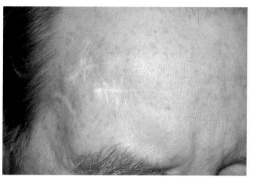

Suture marks on the forehead

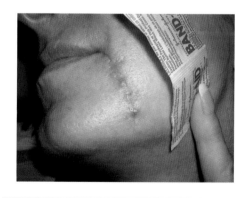

Sterile abscess from a buried suture

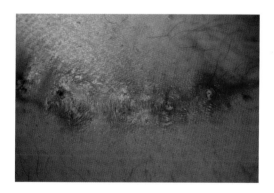

Vicryl sutures 'spitting out'

Hypertrophic scars

Moderate problem scars

Hypertrophic scars are raised, red, and itchy or sore. They occur most often on the chest, upper back, shoulders and breasts. Though more common with full-thickness incisions they can occur after curettage, electrocautery and dermabrasion. Previous hypertrophic scars make further ones more likely. They usually appear around 4–8 weeks following surgery.

Early intervention with steroid injections to the scar may reduce the symptoms and flatten the scar but will not prevent a wide and irregular final outcome.

There is some evidence that silicone preparations can improve symptoms.

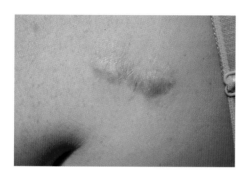

A purple raised scar 6 months after surgery

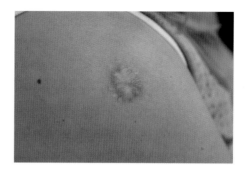

A raised scar 1 year after surgery

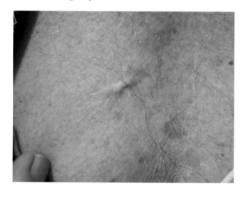

A persistent raised scar on the chest

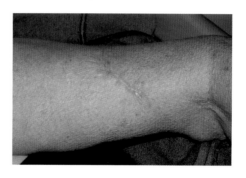

A hypertrophic scar on the upper arm

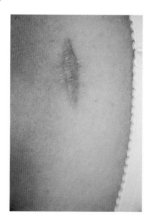

A raised scar on the left shoulder

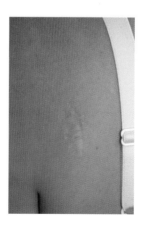

The scar 3 years later, flattened down

Hypertrophic scars

Significant problem scars (keloids)

Huge, painful scarring going beyond the site of original injury is called keloid. Although more common in people of Mediterranean descent and black patients, they may occur in anyone. The earlobes, neck and upper trunk are the most common sites. Treatment is very difficult.

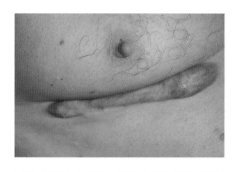

Keloid scar under the breast

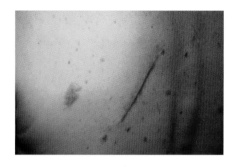

Hypertrophic scar on the back

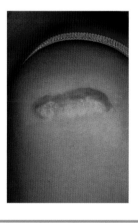

Keloid scar on the shoulder

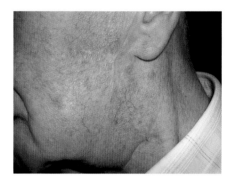

Raised scar on the face

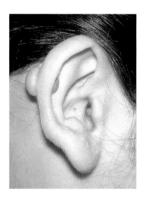

Keloid on ear

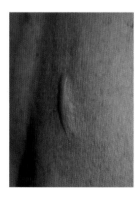

Hypertrophic scar on the back

5

Stretched and indented scars

Stretched scars

Many scars widen over time, and 80% of this occurs in the first 6 months. On the shoulders and upper trunk this may be irrespective of any measures taken to prevent it. In other sites using deep sutures can help to prevent it.

Physically active individuals are more likely to develop stretched scars as are children and young adults.

Indented scars

The problem of indented scars can be overcome to some extent by careful stitching to ensure that the wound edges are a little everted at the end of surgery. Over the days following surgery, there is a tendency for the wound edges to flatten.

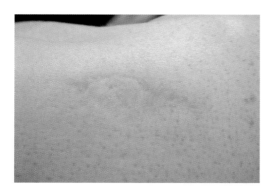

Stretched scar on the shoulder

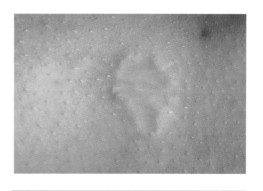

Stretched scar on the back

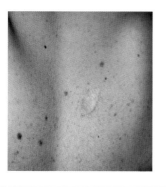

Stretched scar on the back

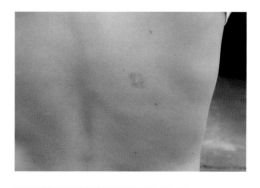

Stretched scar on back

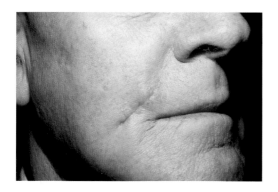

Poor indented scar on the cheek

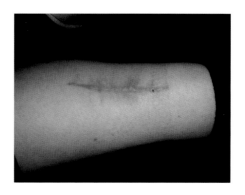

Stretched scar on calf

Allergic reactions

Allergic reactions can often be avoided by taking a careful history. Reactions are possible to the injected local anaesthetic, and they may cause localized swelling, urticaria (hives) or more severe reactions.

Skin cleansing preparations may cause reactions which take several hours to develop. Tincture of iodine used to cause severe reactions, but the more commonly used povodone iodine is a rare cause. Reactions to chlorhexidine are uncommon.

Antibiotic ointments are sometimes put onto wounds with the dressing and several of these can produce sensitivity.

Adhesive tapes are a particular problem and produce a number of reactions, from mild redness and itching to severe reactions with blistering. Even hypoallergenic tapes will produce reactions in susceptible individuals. Mastisol is an adhesive solution also known to cause occasional problems. Tape may also cause a shearing injury to surrounding skin.

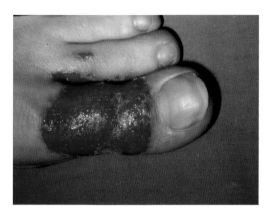

Dermatitis reaction to ointment
under dressing

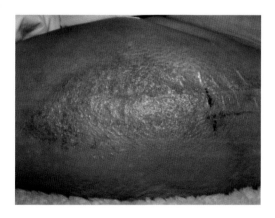

Dermatitis reaction to dressing

Nerve damage

Small nerves are damaged at all operations. The effects are unpredictable and may result in several after effects:

- Mild numbness around the scar
- Numbness in a wide area which may stretch over the scalp, forehead, etc.
- Pain in the immediate area of the scar
- Shooting pains in one direction from the scar
- Unusual feelings of running water, insects, tingling, etc.
- Major damage to a nerve, resulting in weakness of a muscle

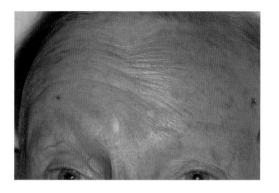

Weakness of forehead muscles

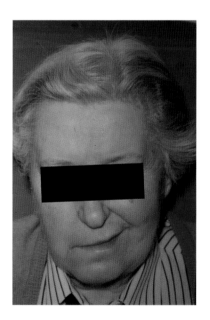

Weakness of facial muscles

Rare healing problems

From time to time wounds heal in a completely unpredictable way. We know that if bare bone is exposed it can be difficult to start the healing process because the tissues cannot establish a blood supply from the underlying bone. Sometimes, however, this same difficulty is encountered when bone has not been exposed at the time of surgery but for some reason it becomes exposed during the healing process.

There are some inherited diseases which are linked to poor healing and unsightly scars. One example is Ehlers–Danlos syndrome.

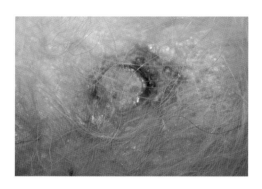

Non-healing wound on the scalp
1 year after surgery

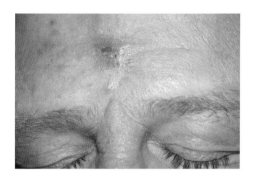

Odd healing 6 months after
surgery

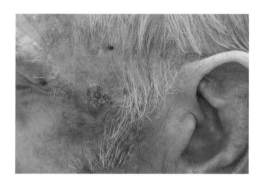

Wet wound 12 weeks after surgery

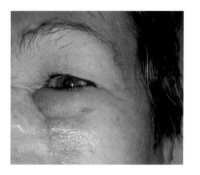

Oedema persisting months after
surgery

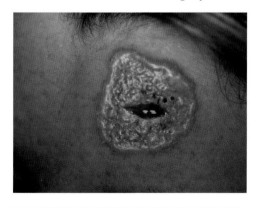

Unexplained healing after
removal of a cyst

Purse-string suture

In some situations it is best to pull the skin together equally from all directions to achieve the best closure. It leaves the wound looking very odd at first with radial corrugations. Good sites for purse-string closure include the temple, the back of the hand and the lower leg.

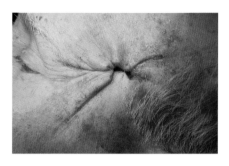

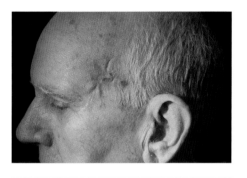

A purse-string suture on the left temple

Within 2 weeks there has been much flattening

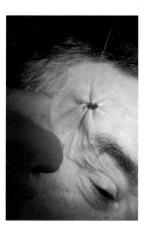

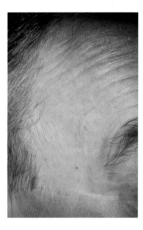

A purse-string suture

The area is well healed after 6 months

Serial excision

Large benign skin lesions can sometimes be best managed by a series of operations. This situation might arise if removal of a lesion, in a single procedure, would result in the need for a skin graft to repair the defect. Removing and suturing only part of the lesion would then allow stretching of the skin over the next few months and the opportunity to remove a further part at a later date.

It is not a technique that can be used for malignant disease because it would be unacceptable to leave some of the diseased tissue behind.

If the shape is irregular it may be necessary to perform excisions at different angles, leading to a bizarre appearance, but if the problem had been severe enough in the first place it may still be a reasonable option. Some tattoos may fall into this category.

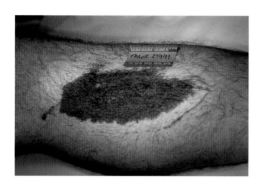

Large pigmented birthmark on leg

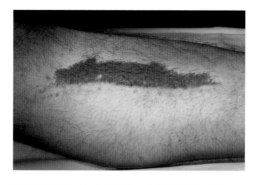

The lesion 8 weeks after the first excision

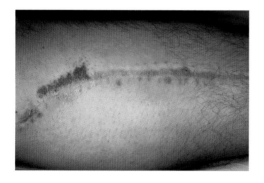

The lesion 8 weeks after the second excision

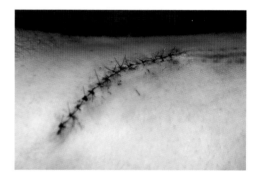

The area after the last part of the lesion has been removed

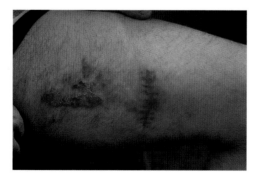

Scars at different angles resulting from serial excision of an irregularly shaped lesion

Flaps

Principles

It may not be possible to close a large defect in the skin by simply drawing the edges together. The principle of a flap is to utilize loose skin from an adjacent area.

The main types of flap are:

- Advancement flaps
- Transposition flaps
- Rotation flaps

The chief problems encountered with flaps are shown on the opposite page. Flaps share most of the same difficulties that can arise with simple excision and primary closure but there are added potential problems related to undermining, interruption of blood supply and the movement of the tissue.

People should be informed before any flap procedure that it is sometimes necessary to do a small second operation at a later date to give the best result. In the case of a pedicle flap, this is always the case, but it should not be considered a failure if removal of a 'dog-ear' or similar is required after a few months.

It is impossible to predict the quality of a scar from skin surgery, including flaps. Healing is an unpredictable event. Sometimes the scars of large flaps fade to become almost imperceptible whereas some smaller flaps may leave imperfect results.

Smoking interferes with healing

Possible complications of flaps

COMPLICATION	REMARKS
Bleeding and haematoma	May occur within hours or be delayed
Infection	Seen most with ulcerated lesions and on the lower limb
Wound separation (dehiscence)	May occur with infection or if the wound is under tension
Suturing complications	Deep stitches may work out. Stitch marks are often seen when stitches are left in for more than 1 week
Hypertrophic scars	Unpredictable unless there is a previous history of the same (see Chapter 5)
Stretched and sunken scars	Quite common on the back or if the wound is under tension
Pigmentary change	More common in skin types 3–6 (see Chapter 5)
Redness and telangiectasia	
Pin cushioning	
Partial take of the flap	
Distortion and 'dog-ears'	More commonly seen in larger excisions
Allergic reactions	Very rare with anaesthetic; reactions to dressings are uncommon (see Chapter 5)
Unexplained poor healing	Rare and unpredictable

Advancement flaps

'Advancement' is the term applied to several types of flap in which the main movement is along one plane. Advancement flaps include:

- Single-sided advancement flaps
- Double-sided advancement flaps
- A-to-T closure
- Island pedicle flaps
- Myocutaneous flaps

Single-sided and double-sided advancement flaps

Pure advancement flaps are simple to conceive but have limited use because the flaps have limited elasticity. In this case the defect is only covered by stretching the flap rather than transferring the tension to an area of lax skin.

In the example opposite (middle row), skin from the lower forehead is stretched to cover a defect on the bridge of the nose. There will be some upward tension and it might slightly elevate the tip of the nose – however, this is often seen as an advantage in elderly people who may have some drooping of the nasal tip.

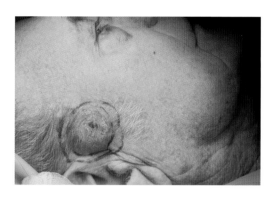

Large lesion in front of the ear

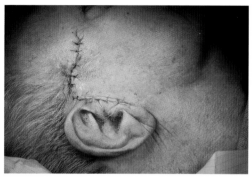

Skin advanced from the jaw and neck

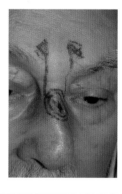

Lesion on the bridge of the nose

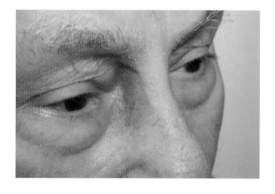

Skin advanced from the forehead

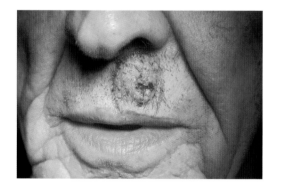

Lesion on the upper lip

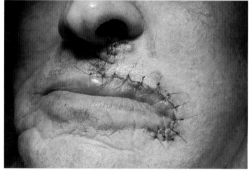

Skin advanced from the cheek

Advancement flaps

A-to-T closure

This method allows the surgeon to avoid cutting across chosen structures such as the eyebrow, lip and hairline. The lesion is removed as an A shape or an inverted A, and by a mixture of chiefly advancement but some rotation, the edges are brought together.

It allows the incision line to lie in a relatively concealed position or in a natural crease and avoids a scar crossing cosmetically sensitive areas such as the vermilion of the lip.

Two single-sided advancements

If two defects, lying close to each other, are sutured separately it is likely that closing each one will increase the tension on the other. In the method illustrated opposite (bottom row), the two defects are joined by an incision that crosses from one side of the top lesion to the opposite side of the bottom lesion. When an attempt is made to suture the top wound it automatically starts to close the bottom wound as well – in other words reducing the tension and thus improving the likelihood of a good outcome.

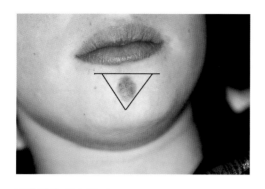

Birthmark on the chin

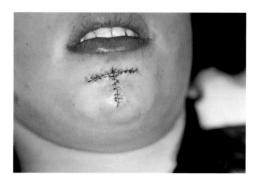

A-to-T advancement closure

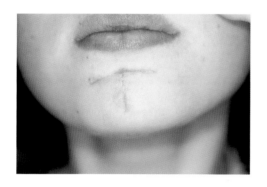

Month after stitch removal

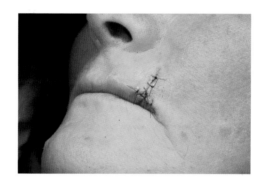

A-to-T closure on the lip

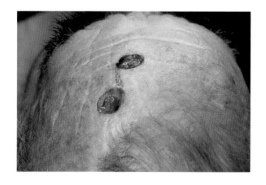

Two defects joined to allow advancement repair

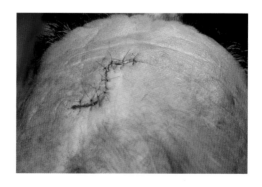

Following repair

Advancement flaps

Island flaps

This method involves freeing up an area of skin on all sides but leaving the base attached to the underlying fat for a blood supply. They can only be used where the underlying tissue is freely moveable (e.g. fatty areas or back of the hand). Generally island flaps have a good blood supply and a low risk of complications. The other chief advantage comes from the way in which the tissue is moved. The defect left behind as the island is advanced is then sewn up in such a way that the island is pushed forward. These so-called 'pushing' flaps are less likely to pull on free edges such as the eyelid, lip, etc.

Good sites for island flaps:

- Cheek
- Back of the hand
- Lateral aspect the upper and lower lip
- Sometimes on the lower leg

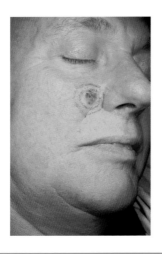

Lesion on the cheek

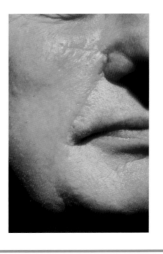

Skin advanced from below
the defect

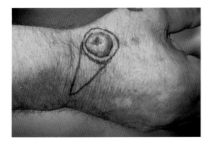

Lesion on the back of the
left hand

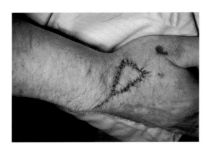

Island advancement

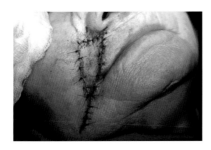

Repair of a lip lesion

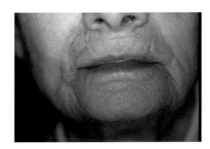

The lip area 6 months later

Transposition flaps

In a transposition flap, tissue is moved from one side of the defect in a swivelling motion. It can be turned through 90° or more but this tends to produce a noticeable hinge effect or a 'dog-ear' at the swivel point. These are commonly used flaps but care must be taken to ensure an adequate blood supply.

Nasolabial flaps

A nasolabial flap is a special example of transposition and allows defects on the lower part of the nose to be filled with cheek skin. It is important to avoid a tenting effect because any bridge across the groove at the side of the nose is easily noticeable. This flap is prone to some pin-cushion effect but with time the appearance tends to improve.

Finger flaps

A finger flap is usually a relatively narrow strip of skin and great attention must be paid not to make it so long that the blood supply is insufficient. It is particularly useful moving skin from the upper eyelid to the lower eyelid and on the helix of the ear.

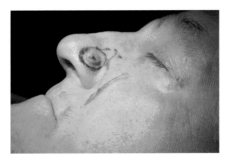

Lesion on the nose

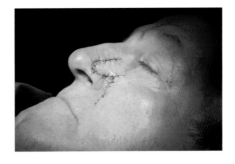

Area after transposition from the cheek

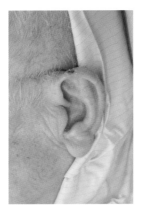

Lesion on the top of the ear

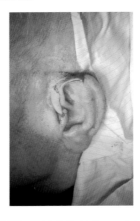

Lesion removed and skin flap raised

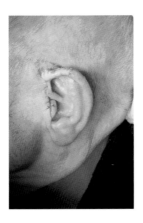

Flap sewn into place

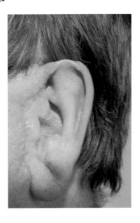

Months later

Transposition flaps

Rhomboid flaps

There are several variations on the same principle. Tissue is raised to one side in such a way that it swivels round into place. If it turns through a big angle there is more of a tendency to produce a raised cone or a 'dog-ear' at the hinge. This can be minimized by selecting flaps with smaller turning angles and wide undermining.

As with all other flaps the chief aim is to get good closure and avoid distorting important structures. If a small corrective procedure is needed at a later date to remove a residual 'dog-ear', the flap should not be deemed a failure.

If the lesion is removed and leaves a circular defect there are many directions from which the flap can be taken. Usually the realistic options are few because of the position and surrounding structures. Sometimes the defect is designed as a rhomboid shape in the first place and the geometry is then a little easier to see. However, the elasticity of skin means that without much trimming, a square flap can be made to fit into a round hole.

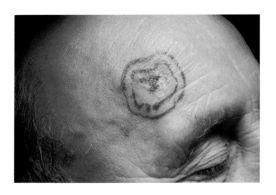

A lesion on the forehead

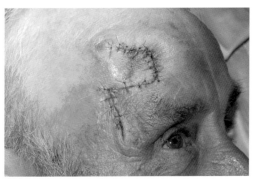

Area after a rhomboid flap

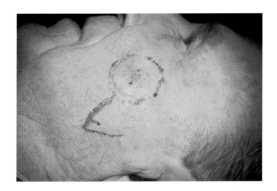

A lesion on the cheek

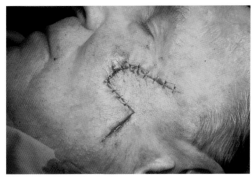

Area after a rhomboid flap

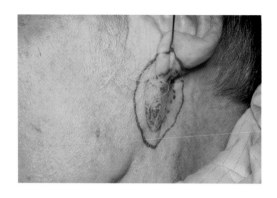

A lesion on the neck

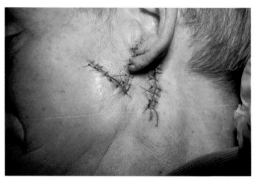

Area after a transposition flap

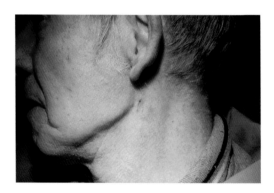

Well-healed area weeks later

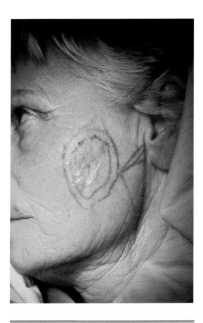

Large lesion on the left
cheek

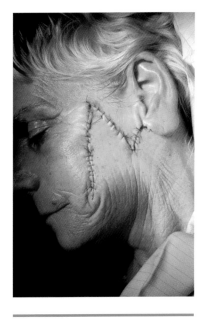

Area after a transposition
flap

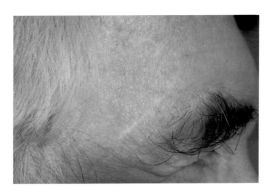

Very well-healed flap

Rotation flaps

A rotation flap is a special type of transposition flap, where a semicircle of tissue is rotated into a circular or triangular defect. The bigger the semicircle is made, the less tension is on the flap and the more likely is success. The tension is sometimes reduced by making a back-cut.

Rotations work well in areas where there is some tissue movement available in all directions. This is particularly the case on the scalp.

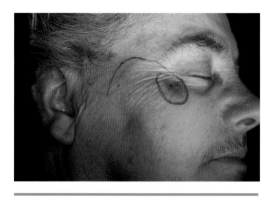

Design of a rotation flap

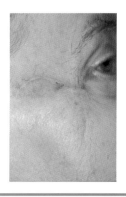

3 months after rotation repair

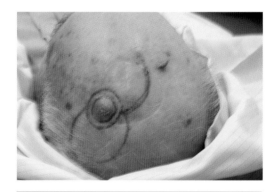

Double rotation on back of scalp

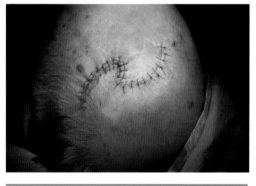

Back of scalp after suturing

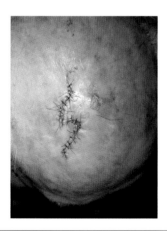

Double rotation on front of scalp

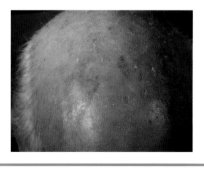

Front of scalp 3 months later

Complications

The frequency with which problems arise after flap repairs is dependent on the site, adherence to postoperative instructions, smoking habits and some unpredictable factors.

The chief problems are:

- Ischaemia or necrosis
- Infection
- Deformity of a free edge (e.g. on the lip)
- Bruising and haematoma
- Dehiscence
- Pin-cushion effect
- Indentation of the scar
- Stretching of the scar
- Hypertrophy of the scar

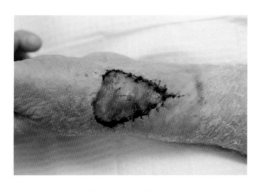

Flap dehiscence at the far end

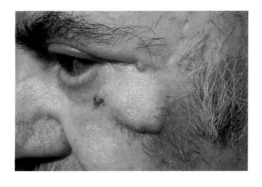

Bulky lower half of flap

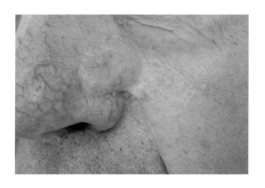

Tenting effect over the crease

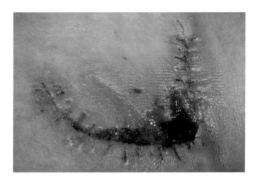

Necrosis at the tip of the flap

Complications

Different sites on the body

There are sections later in the book devoted to some special sites, but there are some overall principles which affect healing.

- The lower limb has poorer healing, and flaps generally must have larger pedicles to prevent ischaemia and necrosis. Equally, infection is more often seen on the lower limb
- Wounds on the back are subject to stretching forces and often heal less well
- Flaps bearing hair are usually on the scalp where the blood supply is good. But if there is ischaemia, the hair follicles can perish

Smoking has an adverse effect on healing

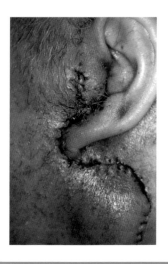

Haematoma under the flap

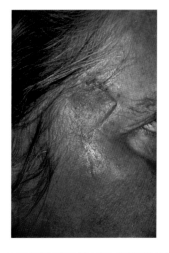

Indented scar line

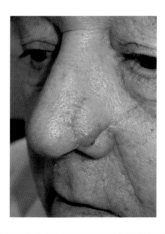

Pin-cushion effect

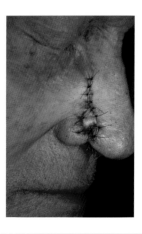

Notch in the alar rim

Complications

Avoiding complications

Whether it is a simple excision, a flap or a graft there are simple principles to follow. Generally it is best to rest, avoid exercise and in particular to keep the affected part relatively still for a few days.

General advice to encourage good healing

- Go home and rest
- Avoid over-exertion and bending down
- Use extra pillows after facial surgery and elevate the leg after lower limb surgery
- Do not drink alcohol or smoke for 48 hours
- Use paracetamol rather than aspirin for pain relief
- If bleeding occurs apply firm pressure for 20 minutes using a clean handkerchief over the dressing

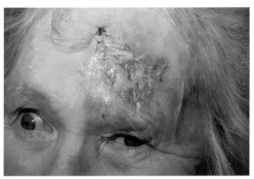

Infection at the surgical site

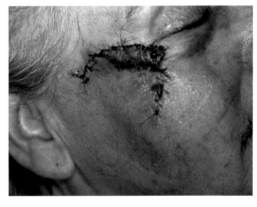

Bowstring effect

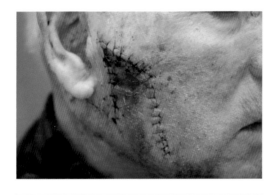

Some necrosis, bruising and infection

Further example of necrosis

Skin grafts

Full thickness grafts

Full thickness grafts are used to cover a defect in the skin when it is not possible to repair it simply by primary closure. Depending on the site it may be quite a small defect, such as on the nose where there is very little spare loose skin. On the other hand it may be possible to close a much bigger defect on the cheek without recourse to a graft.

A full thickness graft, rather than a split skin graft, is used when a superior cosmetic result and greater repair strength are required.

Donor skin

Wherever possible skin is taken with similar features to the recipient site to give the best cosmetic outcome.

Features for matching skin

- Skin thickness
- Surface markings
- Weathering characteristics
- Colour

Suitable donor sites

- Behind or in front of the ear
- Nasolabial fold
- Upper eyelid
- Inner upper arm
- Lower abdominal wall
- Supraclavicular fossa

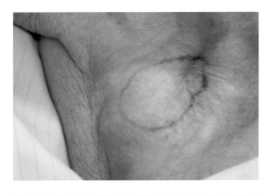

Skin for graft on the right shoulder

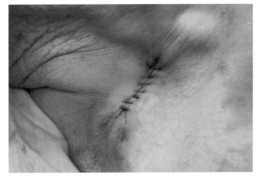

Skin sutures after taking the graft

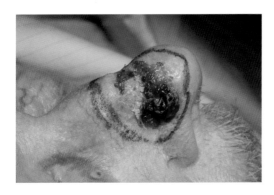

Large lesion on the nose for excision

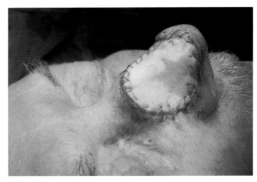

Graft in place (day 1)

Full thickness grafts

Good outcomes

The surgeon will try to achieve the best possible outcome, and several factors will affect the chance of a good result.

- The surgeon will use the best match of donor skin
- The surgeon will ensure good haemostasis
- Antibiotics may be given if infection seems likely
- The patient should take it easy until the dressing is removed
- Smoking should be completely avoided

However there are several factors which are beyond the control of surgeon or patient and these may significantly affect the result.

Unavoidable possible problems that affect outcome

Donor site problems

- Unexpected hair follicles
- Other skin diseases

Recipient site problems

- Previous radiotherapy
- Severe sun damage
- Very deep wound
- Anatomy affected by the excision
- Poor take over exposed bone or cartilage

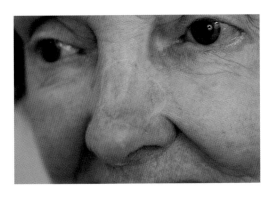

Good result on the nose

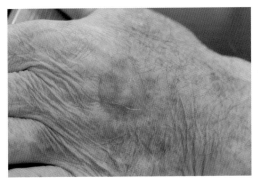

Good result on the hand

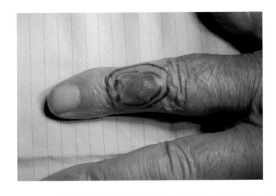

A lesion to be removed on the finger

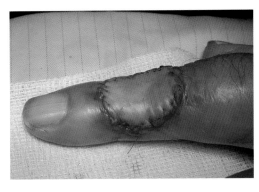

Skin graft in place

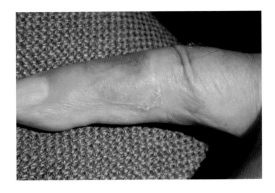

Good result 6 months later

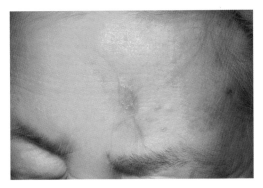

Graft using skin left over from end of the excision

Full thickness grafts

Poor outcomes from complications

Even when everything has been done to maximize the chance of a good result there are some cases that do not go according to plan. Some of the problems that can occur are:

• Wound infection
• Allergic reaction to dressing
• Sunken graft
• Raised and lumpy appearance
• Increased pigmentation
• Decreased pigmentation
• Graft necrosis (partial or complete)
• Pin-cushioning
• Discoloration

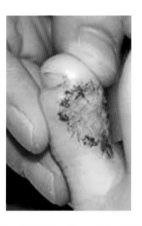

Graft on the toe

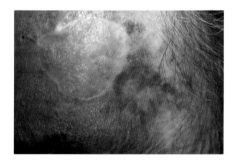

A pale graft on sun-damaged skin

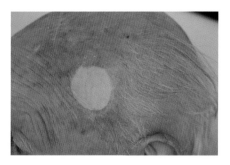

A very pale graft

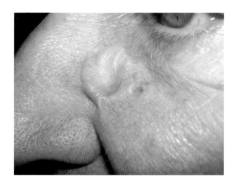

Thickened edge to graft

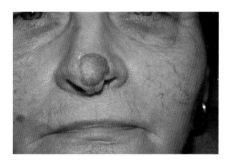

Prominent, raised and discoloured graft

Full thickness grafts

Poor outcomes from complications

Correcting problems

Sometimes people are disappointed with the result of their skin graft at an early stage. It will rarely be helpful to interfere at this stage. Time is the greatest healer and as the months go by grafts tend to become less conspicuous. They flatten and the colour normalizes. Occasionally, with shrinkage a graft begins to pull on a free edge (e.g. the lip, the eyelid or the rim of the nose). This is a considerable problem, and repair is often unsatisfactory. Even an extra-large graft can shrink in this way.

If a graft is bulky and standing proud, it is often helped by injecting a steroid solution into the graft. Some surgeons use dermabrasion in this situation.

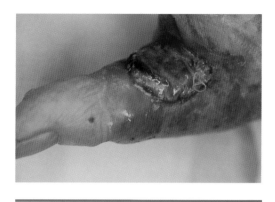

An infected graft

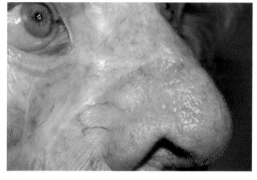

A graft pulling the eyelid

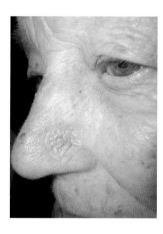

A furrowed, irregular graft

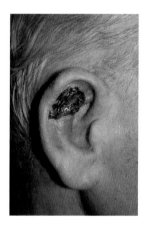

A necrosed graft

Split thickness grafts

A split thickness graft involves slicing off a layer of skin, 0.2–0.45 mm thick, through the dermis, using a hand-held knife or a mechanical dermatome, and leaving behind the lower half of the dermis. This can be done through an Opsite dressing previously applied to the donor skin.

Advantages

- Can be used to cover large areas
- When used to cover a skin cancer wound it allows good visibility of the area for observing possible recurrence of the tumour
- May be less traumatic than a large flap

Disadvantages

- Pain
- Poor healing of the donor site
- Relatively poor cosmetic result and greater graft shrinkage

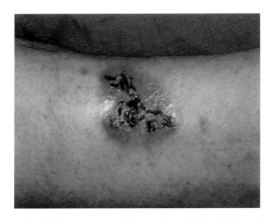

Patch of Bowen's disease

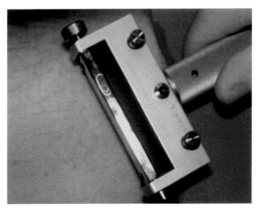

A dermatome

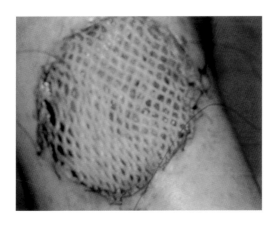

Meshed skin placed on the defect

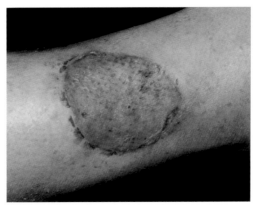

The appearance 1 month later

Split thickness grafts

Meshing, or cutting multiple parallel slits in the graft, allows it to expand when stretched, rather like a fish-net stocking. The gaps fill up with epithelium that has migrated from the surrounding graft. A meshed graft will therefore cover a wider area than a similar sized unmeshed graft, conform to cover an uneven contour (e.g. the ear) and, more importantly and especially on the lower leg, permit exudate to drain through the gaps.

The common donor sites for split-thickness grafts include the upper arm, the upper thigh and the abdominal wall. The donor site can be anaesthetized painlessly and effectively using a eutectic mixture of local anaesthetic, and it heals faster when a calcium alginate or semipermeable, adhesive polyurethane film dressing is used.

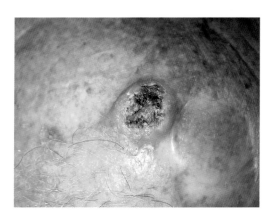

Skin cancer on scalp adjacent to an existing split skin graft

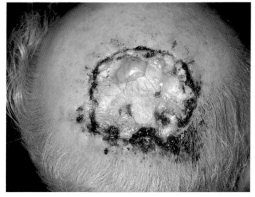

After grafting whole area – moderately health graft site

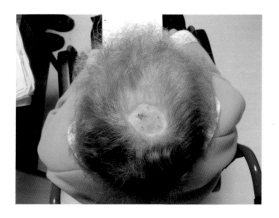

Split-thickness graft after a few years

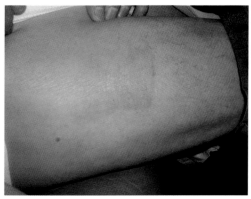

Well-healed donor site

Special sites – the ear

Small lesions

The ear is a complex shape and special approaches are needed to retain that shape wherever possible. Small lesions on the rim or antihelix can be removed and sutured easily. Sometimes there is minimal distortion but it is often not noticeable as both ears are not usually seen at the same time.

In the bowl of the ear there is little room for manoeuvre. The skin is firmly attached to cartilage beneath and does not stretch. Wounds are often left to heal by secondary intention. In this case it is possible to remove small plugs of cartilage and allow skin cells to grow through from the other side to speed up the healing time.

8

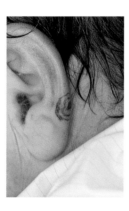

Small lesion on the rim of the helix

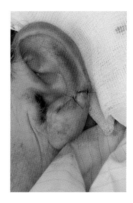

Sutured area after excision of the lesion

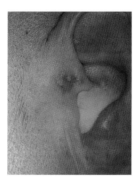

Lesion on crus of ear

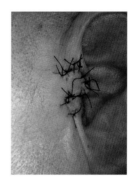

After small flap repair

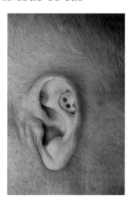

Cartilage plugs removed to aid healing

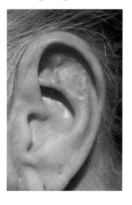

Skin graft to upper part of the ear

Larger lesions

Trimming a small area of the ear

Small areas can be removed by trimming a curved piece from skin and cartilage. The ear becomes a little smaller but retains something like its overall shape.

Some individuals are quite happy to live with an ear whose shape has altered. The ear is not the first thing you look at when meeting people, and indeed the asymmetry does not matter so much as both ears are not normally seen at the same time.

This operation is simple and quick. It has a lower complication rate than more complex procedures such as grafting and skin flaps.

Wedge excision and helical rim advancement

Sometimes it is necessary to remove quite large parts of the ear. Inevitably the ear will become smaller but it can either retain the same shape or retain the same length with a piece carved out of it.

Complications

The cartilage is not elastic, unlike skin. It tends to bend rather than stretch. This makes it more likely for some deformity to arise from these procedures on the ear. Fortunately even a large excision on the ear is unlikely to affect the wearing of spectacles.

Wedge excision and helical rim advancement reduce the circumference of the ear but this is not readily noticeable. Sometimes the join can be obvious when cartilage of different thicknesses are brought together. The ear may fold forward to some extent. Indentation at a join line is called a butterfly deformity.

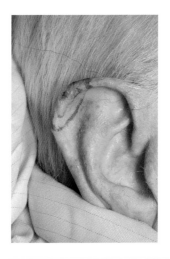

A lesion on the helix

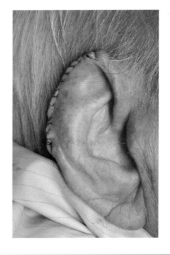

The helix trimmed

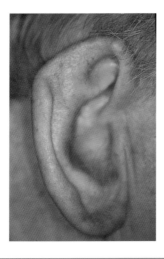

Change in shape after the removal of a lesion

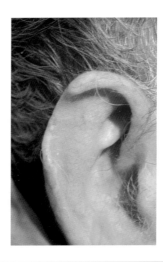

Another example of a change in shape

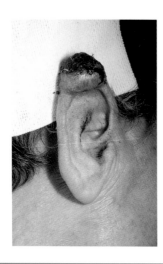

A large lesion on the helix

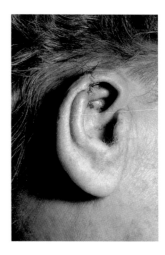

After wedge excision

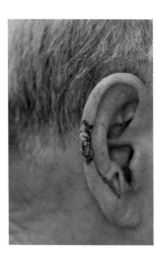

A large lesion on the rim of the helix

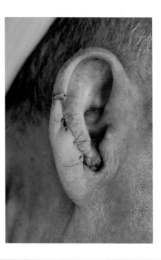

After helical rim advancement

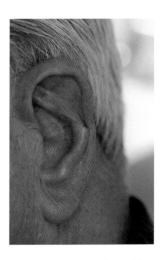

Cartilage of different thickness at a join line

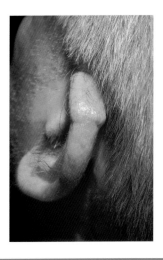

A more marked join line

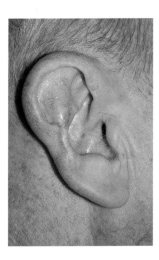

Butterfly deformity

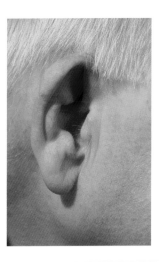

Slight forward folding

Larger lesions

Direct skin-to-skin closure

Direct skin-to-skin closure leaves the length of the ear unchanged but gives an odd shape. Healing tends to be very quick, and the operation is simple – less can go wrong.

On rare occasions it is necessary to remove the entire ear. This sounds horrific but modern prostheses are remarkably lifelike.

Skin grafts

If removal of a large lesion would leave exposed cartilage it may be unwise to allow open healing because of the time it would take to heal, the discomfort and the risk of failure to heal at all. A skin graft should then be considered and they can be applied to the bowl as well as the rim of the ear. It is not easy to keep a dressing, with moderate pressure, applied to the graft for 10 days but it is sometimes necessary.

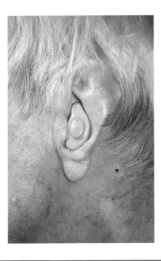

Large excision, left ear

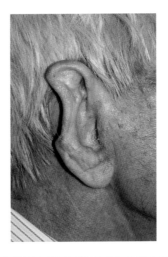

Large excision, right ear

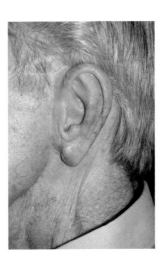

Removal of the entire ear, with prosthesis in place

Pedicle flap from the skin behind the ear

A pedicle flap is another method used to repair a defect on the rim of the ear. It can only be used if there is a large enough area without hair adjacent to the part of the rim to be repaired. The operation takes place in three stages:

- The lesion is excised from the ear
- A flap of skin is elevated from the mastoid area and sewn into the defect
- 2 weeks later the pedicle is cut, the ear is fashioned to look neat, and the area on the mastoid is left to heal by open healing

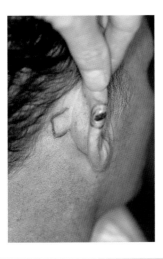

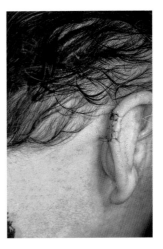

Areas marked for excision and raising pedicle

Pedicle sewn into place

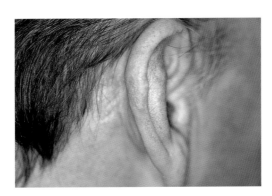

2 months after dividing the pedicle

Special sites – the nose

General principles

The nose has great importance cosmetically because of its central position. Its shape clearly matters to individuals, as evidenced by the number of people who seek some form of nasal reshaping. Surgery on the nose is therefore accompanied, more than for most other areas, by anxiety that it might result in deformity, asymmetry or an adverse result.

It is true that there is less room for manoeuvre than in many other sites. This means that the doctor must be aware of all the possible methods of treatment to advise on the best approach to deal with a particular problem.

Special problems

When considering surgical repair, whether by primary closure, flaps or grafts, there are a number of special features which need to be taken into account:

- Nasal skin is thick – grafts may not sit well
- Nasal skin has more sebaceous glands than surrounding skin
- Nasal skin has a greater tendency to pin-cushion defect than most areas
- Small tension on the free alar rim can produce an unsightly effect
- The alar groove is cosmetically important, and tenting across it is a problem
- Tension on the distal third can affect the airway

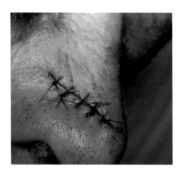

After excision of a lesion on the nose

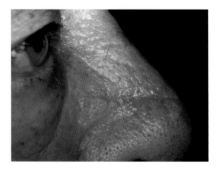

The area 2 months later

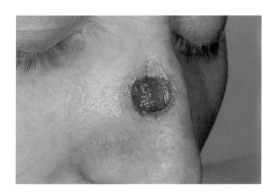

Nose after removal of a tumour

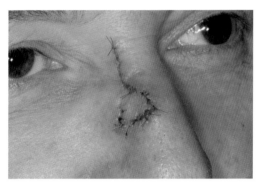

Nose after a rhomboid flap

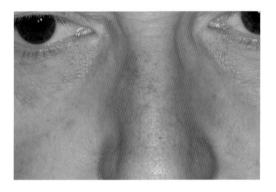

The area months later

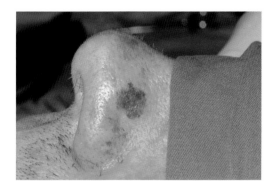

A large lesion on the left side of the nose

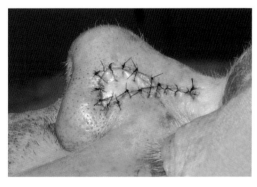

Myocutaneous flap

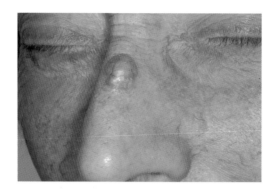

Basal cell carcinoma on the nose

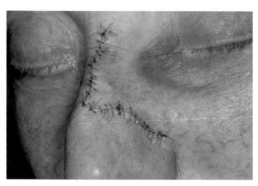

The area following a rotation flap

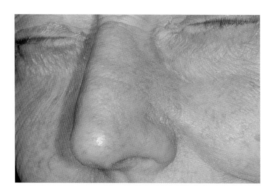

The area months later

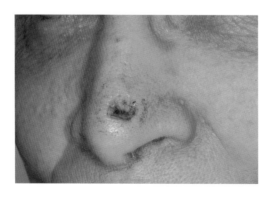

Defect on the nose

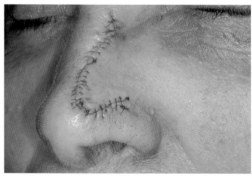

A rotation flap

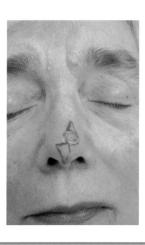

One type of nasal tip excision

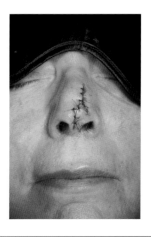

After excision and repair

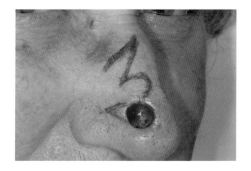

Defect on the nose

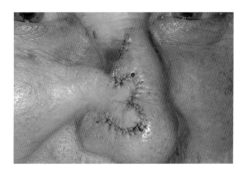

After bilobed repair

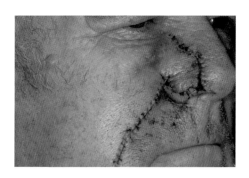

A nasolabial flap in place

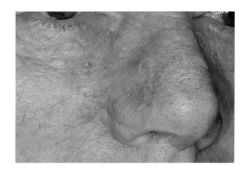

A matured flap

Complications

The thick, sebaceous skin, prominent position and subtle shape and curves of the nose make it liable to cosmetic problems after surgery. As with many other areas of the skin, it is difficult to predict the likely cosmetic outcome of a procedure; sometimes after extensive repairs there can be little to see whereas sometimes even small excisions can leave a prominent mark.

Chief problems

* Blunting of the angle in the alar crease, which can occur easily after any form of repair in that area
* Elevation of the alar rim
* Mismatch of skin texture and thickness with flaps and grafts
* Pinching of the nasal tip
* 'Ski-tip' deformity

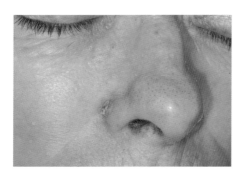

Depressed scar at the alar crease

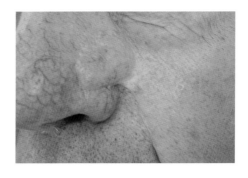

Nasolabial tenting

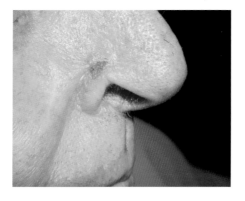

Raised alar rim

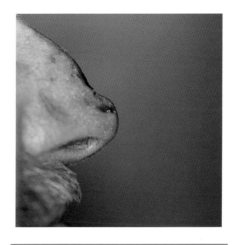

'Ski-tip' shape to the end of the nose

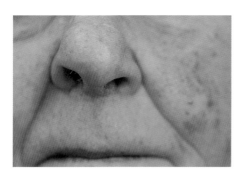

Asymmetry of the nostrils

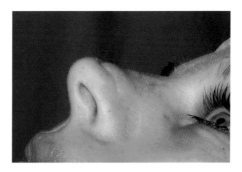

Pin-cushion effect

Special sites – the lips

General principles

The lips are cosmetically very important and are vital for speaking, eating and non-verbal communication. They are formed in part by skin (dry) and mucosa (red and wet). They have a rich blood supply and a complex system of muscles underneath to form many different positions. It is important that the lips should be able to seal completely, otherwise dribbling may result. Small irregularities are readily visible. The upper lip is particularly challenging in this regard because it has subtle curves, hollows and mounds, which may be lost after a repair.

Chief problems

Main problems after surgery:

- Scars crossing the vermillion are often noticeable
- Any distortion of the free edge can look like a snarl
- Increased risk of hypertrophic scars
- Stitches can be irritating on the mucosal surface

Small lesions

Small lesions on the lip may be removed and stitched easily side-to-side, usually in a vertical direction. However, if there is any tension causing distortion then a small skin flap or graft may be preferred. Alternatively, small defects of the mucosal lip can be left to heal spontaneously with good results. It is best to avoid crossing the vermilion if possible.

As with all other areas, if there is a residual distortion after surgery then a second corrective procedure may be suggested at a later stage to improve the appearance.

Larger lesions

Larger lesions may require a skin flap or graft to repair the defect. A wedge of full thickness of lip may be removed, then the two sides realigned and stitched together. This can result in a smaller, tighter mouth but with simple stretching exercises it becomes looser in time.

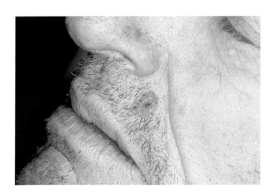

Lesion on the lip

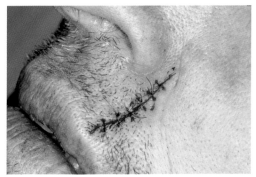

Area after excision of the lesion

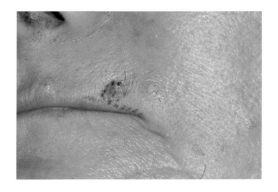

Lesion on the vermilion border

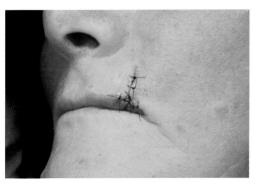

Area following surgery with a small A-to-T closure

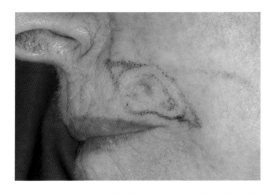

Large lesion on the upper lip

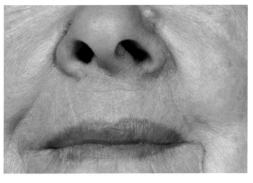

Area 5 months after primary closure

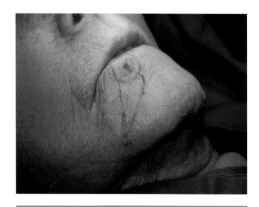

Lesion on the lower lip

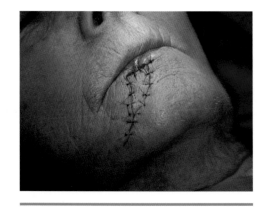

Area after island flap repair

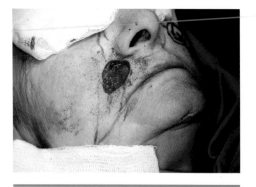

Large lesion on the upper lip

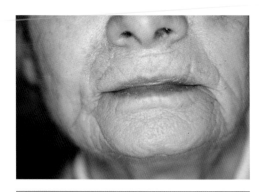

Area after island flap repair

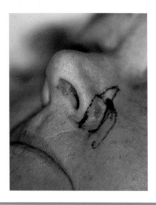

Lesion at the junction of the nose
and the lip

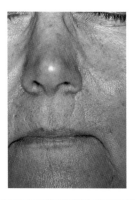

Area after rotation flap

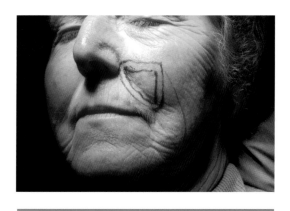

Before flap

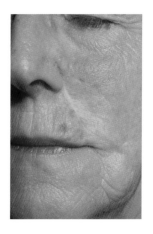

2 years later

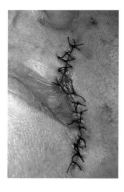

Immediately after surgery

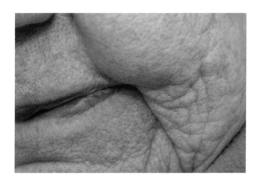

2 years later

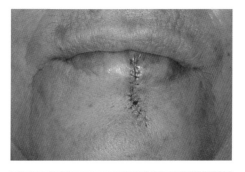

Excision through the skin and mucosa

Poor results

The lip is cosmetically a very sensitive area. Even small irregularities can be obvious. Pulling on the vermilion border is disfiguring and any unevenness in the line of the vermilion is noticeable. Great care is taken to try and avoid these problems but sometimes scarring is unpredictable.

As with all other areas of skin there is a possibility of hypertrophic scarring, and it is slightly more common on the lip than many other sites. Wherever possible the incision lines are made in the natural creases or along the vermilion border. Although the crease from the nose to the corner of the mouth is a good site to place the scar, it must be done with care because it can be very obvious, like a railway track, if the scar lies parallel to the crease rather than in it.

Serious sun damage to the lower lip produces crusty, white areas with a high risk of malignant change. The entire lower lip mucosa can be removed and fresh tissue from within the mouth undermined and pulled forward to reline the lip. This usually gives a better result than trying to remove only the most affected parts.

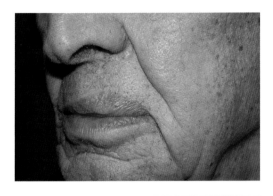

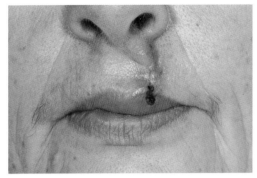

Pulling on the vermilion following surgery

A large defect repaired, but there is some distortion and the wound is not completely healed

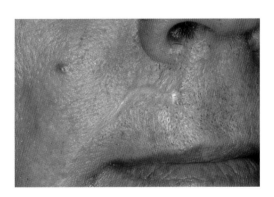

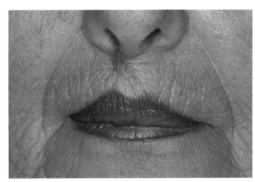

Thickened scar on upper lip

Tethering after open wound healing

Special sites – the eye

General principles

Every effort is made to plan a repair which will not affect the function of this special site and also minimize the change in appearance. The lacrimal gland and the tear ducts are crucial in their function of keeping the eye moist. The eyelid skin is loosely attached to the structures underneath, and this results in very easy and often pronounced swelling and bruising. The eye may close completely after the surgery.

Small lesions

Small lesions near the eye may be removed and stitched easily side-to-side. The closure is in a vertical direction to avoid ectropion.

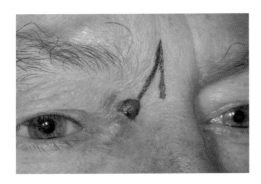

Small flap for a medial defect

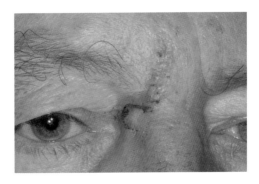

Area after repair

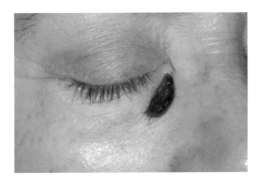

A defect on the lower eyelid

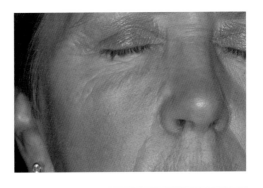

Area after advancement repair

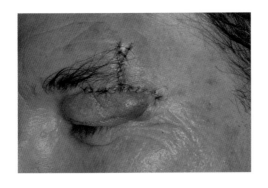

Immediately after closure on the eyebrow

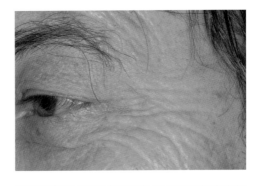

Area 4 months later

General principles

Larger lesions

Larger lesions usually require a skin flap or graft to repair the defect. The same principles apply to large defects as to small ones, with the most important being avoidance of any pulling effect on the lower lid.

The snap test refers to a simple test in which the lower lid is pulled down and then watched as it returns to its normal position. There should be a rapid return, owing to the complex anatomy and elasticity of the tissues specifically designed to make this happen. At the mid-point in an operation when the key sutures have been put into place, it is a good idea to try the snap test – often with the patient sitting upright so that gravity is working against the lid. If it does not move back into place there should be reconsideration of the closure technique.

Immediately after surgery there can be a worrying appearance of the lid bulging out and not being in direct contact with the globe. This is usually due to tissue swelling and the volume of local anaesthetic that has been injected. It should settle within 1–2 days. For weeks after surgery there is a tendency for scarring and retraction to occur, and ectropion may develop, disappointingly, at this stage.

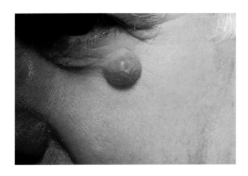

Tumour on the lower eyelid

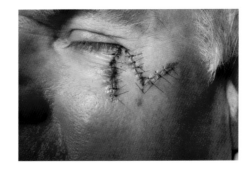

Area after flap repair

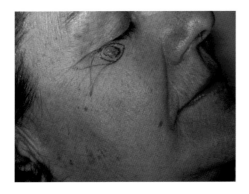

Lesion on the lower eyelid

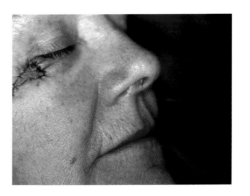

Area after island flap repair

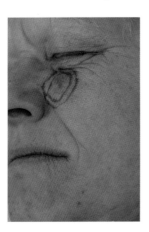

Large lesion below the eye

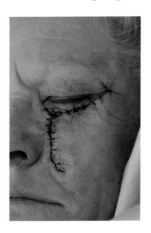

Flap angled to avoid downward
tension on the eyelid

Complications

Ectropion

The lower lid is readily affected by quite mild pulling forces with a resulting downward deformity, called ectropion. If there is tension on the lower eyelid after surgery, especially if the eyelid was a bit loose beforehand, then the lower lid can be pulled down (ectropion), causing excessive watering. This may correct itself in time or it may need a second surgical procedure to correct it.

Oedema

Rarely, swelling under the eye can persist over a much longer period of time, owing to scar formation blocking the draining lymph channels.

Open wound healing

Open wound healing is discussed in more detail in Chapter 13, but the method can be utilized with benefit around the eye if cases are chosen with care. Small, shallow surgical defects of the lower eyelid and symmetrical defects at the inner corner of the eye may be left to heal by themselves with good resultant appearance and no impairment of function.

Eyebrows

Surgery on or above the eyebrows can result in damage to some hair follicles and shortening of the brow. Raising or an uneven eyebrow after removal of bigger lesions is a possibility. Removing lesions at the glabella can bring the eyebrows slightly closer together.

Difficult skin cancers

Some really difficult lesions may require wider and deeper surgery, and in such cases skin grafts and flaps are used for repair. The problems associated with this type of surgery are:

- The usual problems that can be seen elsewhere
- Ectropion, even if the repair initially seems to have worked well
- Damage to the tear-producing or collecting apparatus, which can result in a dry eye and may necessitate the use of artificial tears in future

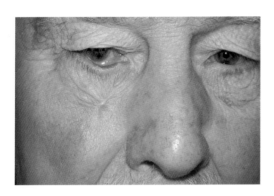

Ectropion after surgery

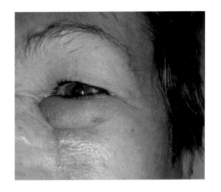

Persistent oedema months after surgery

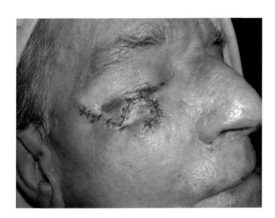

Immediately after surgery

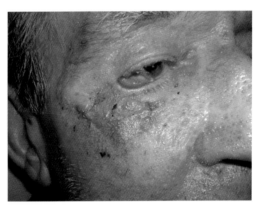

Ectropion due to contraction

Special sites – the nails

Procedures on the nails

A number of problems affect the nail and the tissues around it. The type of biopsy recommended will depend on the primary tissue involved. In the diagram opposite the numbers illustrate:

1 The relationship between components of the nail unit and the underlying bone.
2 Tissue taken at the free end of the nail to investigate discoloration and thickening.
3 An area of the nail bed that could be biopsied after removal of the nail plate.
4 Incisions made in the skin to allow reflection of the cuticle and nail fold.
5 Punch biopsy taken at the base of a narrow pigmented band.
6 Larger horizontal biopsy taken for a wider pigmented band.

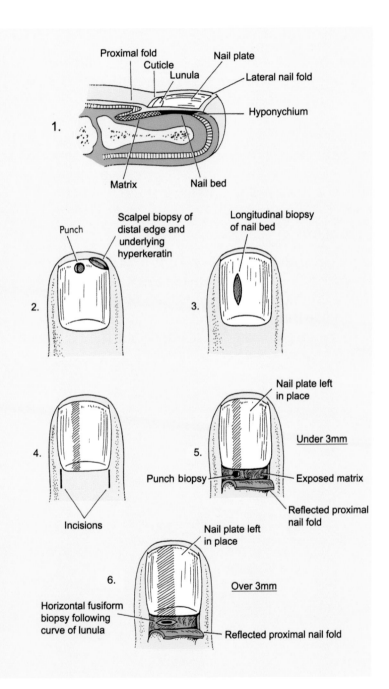

1. Proximal fold — Cuticle — Lunula — Nail plate — Lateral nail fold — Hyponychium — Matrix — Nail bed

2. Punch — Scalpel biopsy of distal edge and underlying hyperkeratin

3. Longitudinal biopsy of nail bed

4. Incisions

5. Nail plate left in place — Under 3mm — Punch biopsy — Exposed matrix — Reflected proximal nail fold

6. Nail plate left in place — Over 3mm — Horizontal fusiform biopsy following curve of lunula — Reflected proximal nail fold

Problems at the end of the nail

Samples may be taken from the end of the nail for suspected fungal infection. Clippings or soft debris from under the nail are then sent to the laboratory for examination.

Painful hard areas of keratin can form, particularly under the great toenail, in which case it may be due to tight-fitting footwear. However, there are other causes, and it may be necessary to take a punch biopsy with or without the need to clip back the nail a little.

Nail bed problems

All of the tissue under the nail, except for the half-moon, is called nail bed. Many diseases can affect this area, and if it becomes necessary to take a biopsy the nail must be removed to expose the problem. Ideally it is only the least amount necessary that is removed. At a later stage more extensive surgery may be needed, but the first priority is to reach a diagnosis.

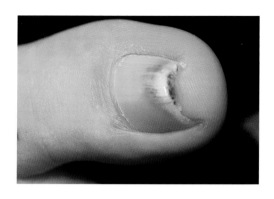

Painful area under the free edge of the nail

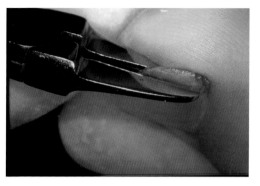

Nail clipping to identify fungus infection

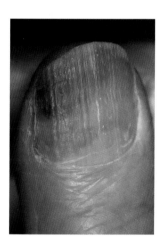

Problem affecting the nail bed

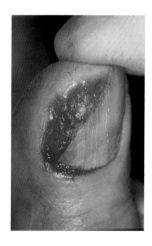

Biopsy possible after the nail has been trimmed back

Nail bed problems

It is essential to visualize the nail bed if there is a disease process beneath the nail plate. A small lesion can sometimes be dealt with by opening a small window in the nail plate using a punch biopsy. The disc of nail is replaced at the end of the procedure and will tend to reattach to the nail bed, but a small piece of tape can be kept in place for a few days if necessary.

Generally it is not necessary to remove the entire nail plate, and it is more comfortable after surgery if most of the plate is left intact. If the problem is to one side then a piece of nail can be taken from that side.

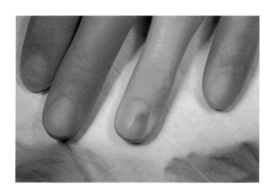

Glomus tumour under the nail

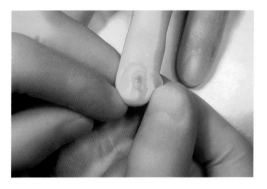

Part of the plate reflected to expose the lesion

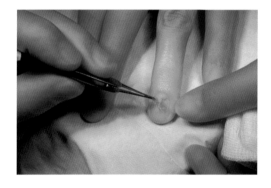

Glomus tumour removed

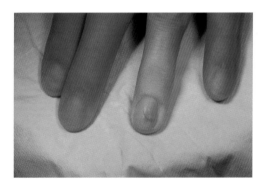

Nail plate replaced

Nail matrix problems

In-growing toe nail

Because nail is made by the matrix it is possible to stop production of nail at the edge by destroying a small part of the matrix. This is usually done by clipping out a length of nail at the edge and then applying a chemical such as phenol or sodium hydroxide to the exposed matrix.

Tumours growing from the matrix

Sometimes a small growth appears from the matrix area; it may also arise from the skin of the proximal fold, or from a combination of the two. The proximal fold is laid back after incisions are made at the two sides. After the tumour has been removed, two stitches are usually sufficient to repair the skin.

Pigmented longitudinal streaks

There is always concern that such a streak might represent a malignant lesion developing in the matrix. The abnormal cells will be found there, so the proximal fold must be laid back to expose the relevant tissue. A punch biopsy from the base of the streak is taken.

Complications of matrix biopsy

- The pain can be unpleasant
- Bleeding
- A permanent groove in the nail plate may arise, especially if the biopsy is large. In an extreme example there could be a split in the nail, which is very awkward

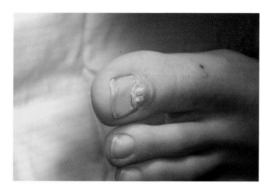

Fibrokeratoma under the nail

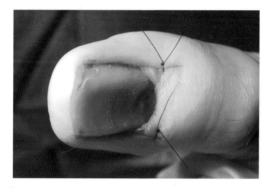

Area after removal

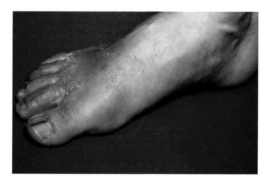

Pigmented streak necessitates biopsy of the matrix

Longitudinal biopsy

It may not be clear whether a dystrophy arises in the bed or the matrix. Sometimes a tumour may extend across both. Here the technique is to remove a piece of tissue that includes all the elements – skin, nail plate, nail bed, matrix. The specimen must go down to the bone. Ideally this is done in the lateral nail folds to avoid a cosmetic problem. If this is not possible then the biopsy should be 3 mm or less in diameter, otherwise it will produce a permanent defect over the length of the nail.

Postoperative care

The finger tends to be very sore after this procedure. The limb should be elevated for 1–2 days. The dressing is changed daily until blood staining ceases. If the lesion appeared to be infected then antibiotics are often prescribed at the time of surgery. Certainly postoperative pain persisting beyond a few days should be adjudged as indicating an infection in most cases.

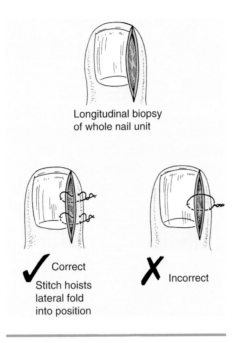

Longitudinal biopsy
of whole nail unit

✓ Correct

Stitch hoists
lateral fold
into position

✗ Incorrect

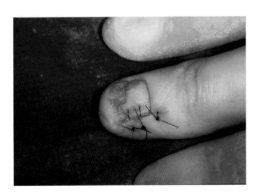

Immediately after longitudinal
biopsy

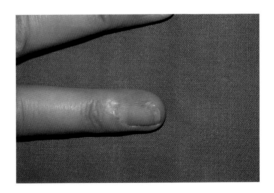

Months after longitudinal biopsy

Open wound healing, partial closure and lattice closure

Theory of open wound healing (natural healing)

In nature many wounds heal without the aid of surgical intervention. Superficial wounds such as grazes always heal in this way. There is a skill in deciding which deeper wounds will heal well if they are left open or only partly closed. The careful use of this approach has been documented more over the past 50 years and has been described in general surgery and orthopaedic surgery as well as in dermatology and plastic surgery.

Why use open healing?

If it is not possible to close a wound easily, without distortion or undue tension, there are several alternatives, which include skin grafts, flaps and open wound healing or partial closure.

The advantages of open healing are:

- It is simple and avoids skin grafts or more complex surgery
- It is quick which for some people in poor health is an advantage

- The cosmetic results can be superior to other methods in selected cases
- It has a low complication rate in properly selected cases
- It is usually painless throughout
- Allows operator to check that all the tumour has been removed. If the report shows incomplete removal one week later it is easy to go back to remove some more tissue

Which areas give best results?

The cosmetic result of wounds healed by secondary intention varies according to anatomic site:

- Often excellent in concave surfaces of the nose, eye, ear and temple
- Usually fair to good on convex surfaces of the nose, oral lips, cheeks and chin, and helix of the ear. Superficial wounds tend to be heal well, but deep wounds heal with depressed or hypertrophic scars acceptable only to some patients
- Often acceptable on the forehead, antihelix and eyelids and on the remainder of the nose, lips and cheeks

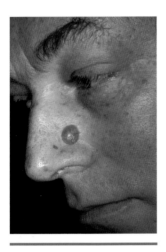

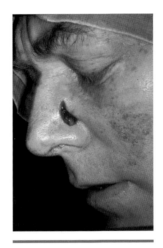

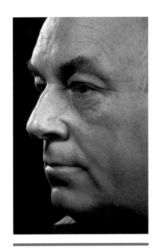

Lesion before removal   Partial closure   Final healing

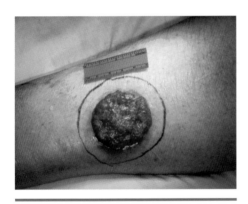

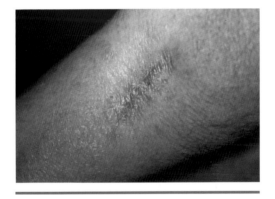

Large lesion on the calf   Area healed after open healing

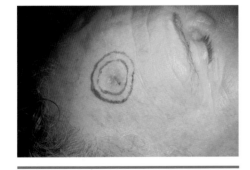

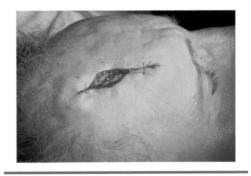

Lesion on the scalp   Partial closure of scalp lesion

Special situations

Hair-bearing scalp

The ability of an open wound to contract is helpful on the scalp because it pulls the hair back together. A skin graft would leave a hairless area and hair-bearing flaps have some limitations.

This approach can be used to significant effect but it demands careful explanation to the patient. A large wound left open in the scalp is difficult to dress and the discharge during the healing phase will be a nuisance. However, as the contractive stage of healing develops, the wound starts to shrink quite quickly and the adjacent hair bearing skin edges are brought together.

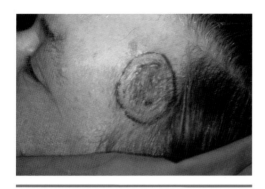

Lesion on the temple

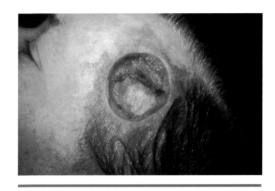

Open wound

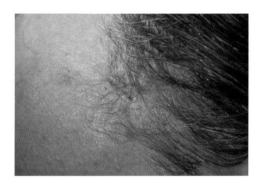

Complete healing – hair restored

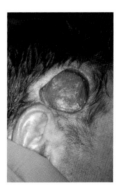

Large open wound

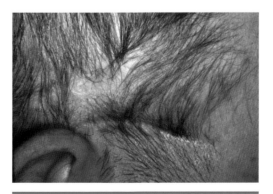

Excellent healing

Special situations

Inner canthus

Wounds in the corner of the eye adjacent to the nose can heal very well. It is important that the wound lies in a position approximately 50% above and 50% below the palebral fissure. Much below this will tend to pull down on the lower lid as it contracts and will cause distortion of the upper lip. A risk in this site is the development of a bowstring effect across the canthus sometimes called an epicanthic fold.

Problems with open healing

- Healing can be slower than expected (i.e. dressings on for longer)
- If the wound goes very deep (e.g. to the bone) then healing can be a problem
- Near a free edge the wound can pull and distort as it contracts
- Hypopigmented scarring is common

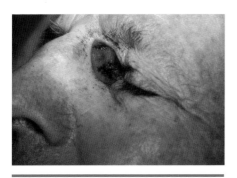

Open wound at the canthus

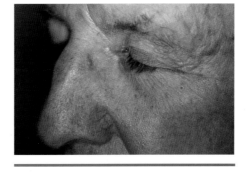

Wound healed without stitches

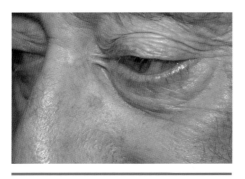

Wound pulling on corner of eye

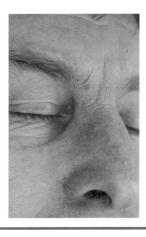

Poor result from open healing

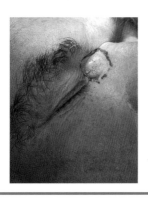

Prior to surgery

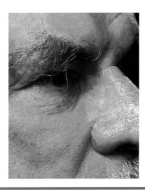

Good result from open healing

Lattice closure

Lattice closure is another method of partial closure. The principle is that several small wounds will heal at the same pace and therefore speed up overall healing compared with one big wound. The idea is the same as making lattice pastry, and a series of slits allow the tissue to be pulled closer together. Initially it looks a little odd but the end result should be compared with the appearance of a skin graft, which might well have been the only other method of closure.

Healing on convex surfaces gives less good, and generally the lower limb gives less good results.

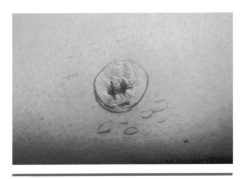

Lesion on the calf

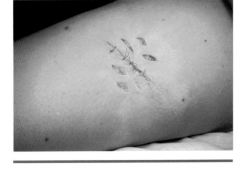

Lattice closure

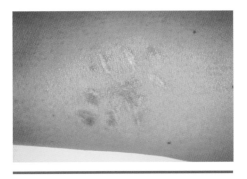

Area 6 months later

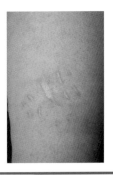

A further example of results from lattice closure

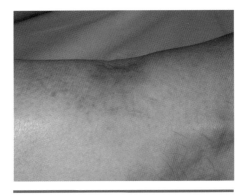

Less good result on the shin

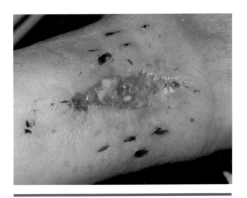

Infected area with slow healing

Wound dressings

Dressings

The surgical procedure completed, a dressing will usually be applied. Verbal and written advice will be given on features of complications to look out for and how and when to change the dressing and clean the wound. If sutures have been used instructions will be given on when these need to be removed.

Wound care and the dressing are important parts of the healing process to ensure a low rate of complications and a good cosmetic outcome. In 1958 it was observed that blisters heal faster if left unbroken. In 1962 it was observed that occlusion of wounds with polythene more than doubled the healing rate in pigs. Moist wound healing has been shown to be 40% faster than air-exposed wound healing, and therefore the common lay advice to 'leave it open to the air to dry' is not the best advice. Epidermal migration is facilitated by moist conditions and the absence of crust. A moist, occlusive dressing with regular changes to allow cleaning and removal of any crust encompasses all these observations and is the ideal environment for healing.

A good surgical wound dressing should:

- Provide a moist environment
- Wick ooze and exudates away from the wound
- Provide protection from infection and foreign material
- Aid in haemostasis
- Limit motion in surrounding tissues
- Cushion the wound against mechanical trauma

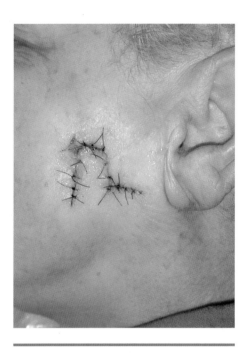

Optional antibiotic ointment

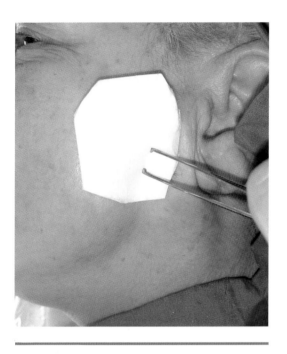

Non-adherent layer

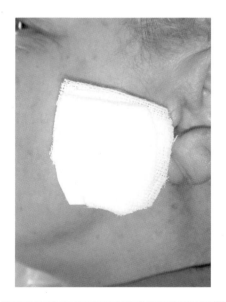

Absorbent and contouring layer

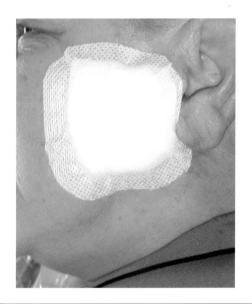

Securing layer

The ideal dressing

The ideal dressing will therefore comprise some or all of the following:

- An ointment (e.g. antibiotic, petrolatum)
- A non-adherent, non-adhesive contact layer
- An absorbent layer (e.g. gauze pads)
- A contouring layer (e.g. gauze pads, dental rolls)
- A securing layer (e.g. tape, tubular bandage, elasticated bandages)

The first 48 hours after the procedure are the most important. If the dressing is saturated by exudate or blood it should be changed. A clean surgical wound does not need daily dressings. When changing dressings care should be taken not to disrupt re-epithelialization.

Sometimes a simpler, lighter dressing is quite adequate, e.g. suture strips may be used as the dressing. Some surgeons will use simple micropore dressing and there is a skin-coloured one available.

If more pressure is required, because of the risk of bruising, firm pressure can be achieved with multiple strips of adhesive tape or the 'butterfly' elastoplast.

Minimalist dressing

Although there is good reason to protect fresh wounds, there is a school of thought that minimal intervention is best. Simple wounds closed primarily can be left open or with a simple micropore or similar covering. It is best to avoid friction on clothing, exposure to environmental irritants such as dust and long soaks in water at an early stage. However, there is no evidence that washing the wound in clean water at an early stage has any deleterious effect.

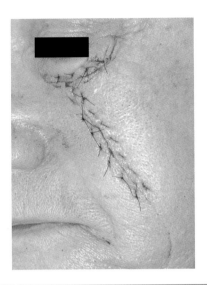

Cheek the wound after the first few days

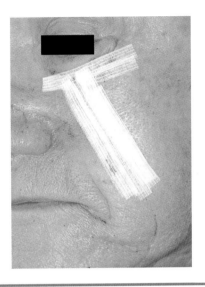

Simple strips applied

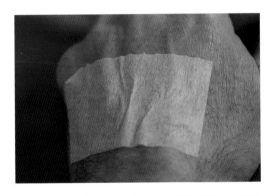

Simple micropore dressing

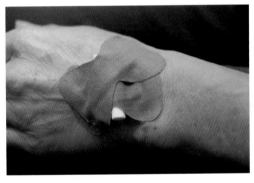

Firmer pressure using butterfly elastoplast

Specialized sites

Skin grafts

Skin grafts must be immobilized for 7–10 days, and there are several ways of achieving this. A tie-over bolster dressing is very popular, but mouldable Aquaplast and multiple applications of stretchy adhesive tape are also used.

Digits

Digits need to be protected because they are readily knocked in every-day life. They require a tubular bandage. Improved healing and reduced pain can be achieved in the hand by using a sling, but elevating the foot of course means very limited mobility after operations in that area.

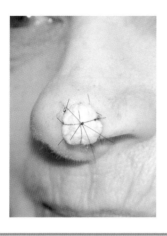

Tie-over dressing to a graft

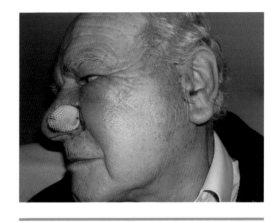

Aquaplast graft dressing

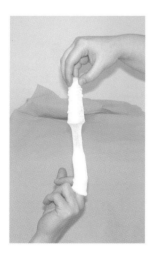

Tubular dressing to a digit

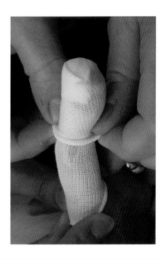

Final appearance of tubular dressing

Specialized sites

Lower limb

The lower leg has a tendency towards impaired circulation and slower healing. It is helpful to measure the ankle–brachial Doppler index before surgery and, if it is satisfactory, apply a graduated compression support as a final dressing layer.

Scalp

The scalp, forehead and ears are very vascular and if bleeding has been a problem during the surgery, a pressure bandage is very helpful. Care must be taken to pad the ear carefully with a contouring layer both behind and in front of the ear, and not to use excessive pressure, or else skin and cartilage necrosis will result.

Dressing complications

- Excessive pressure can cause blistering, ulceration, cartilage necrosis and flap or graft failure
- Insufficient pressure can allow bleeding and haematoma
- Excessive occlusion may promote bacterial overgrowth
- Inappropriate contact layer can cause pain and bleeding with dressing changes
- Medicaments or adhesives can cause allergic contact dermatitis

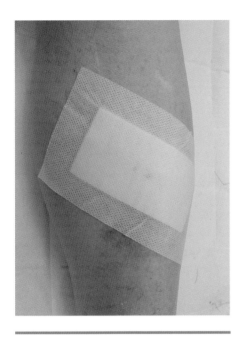

Primary dressing to a leg wound

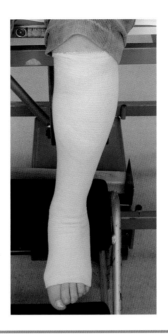

Complete leg support

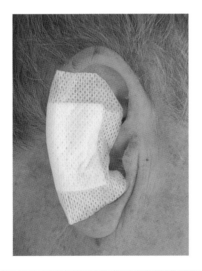

Primary dressing to the ear

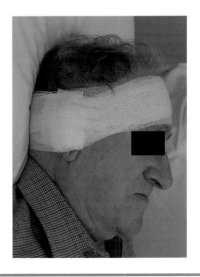

Good support for ear wounds
and other head wounds

Topical therapy

Imiquimod

Imiquimod cream is used to boost the body's natural defences against abnormal cells. The chief uses on the skin are for actinic keratosis and basal cell carcinoma. Treatment is usually accompanied by a vigorous skin reaction with crusting, redness and a stinging or burning sensation. The cream must be applied over several weeks and in visible sites this can be a cosmetic problem. Success rates for superficial basal cell carcinoma are around 85% 'quite good' and the final cosmetic result tends to be 'excellent'. Nodular basal cell carcinomas are cured in only around 65% of cases, less frequently and the treatment is up to 12 weeks.

A few people suffer mild flu-like symptoms during treatment.

Advantages

- Simple cream application
- Useful for those who fear surgery or who might have bleeding problems

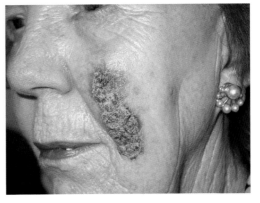

Basal cell carcinoma before treatment with imiquimod

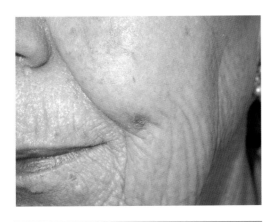

Area after 6 weeks' treatment

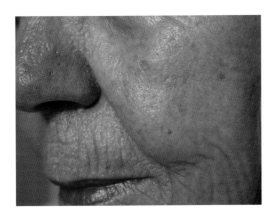

Area 18 weeks after stopping treatment

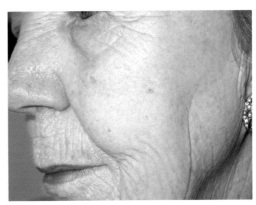

Area 1 year later

Imiquimod

Disadvantages

- Requires 6 weeks' application for thin lesions
- Requires 12 weeks' application for nodular lesions
- Some sites are inaccessible if there is no assistance for application
- Often causes marked inflammation
- Cure rates are not very high
- Causes flu-like symptoms in some people

Effectiveness

There are no very long-term studies but it seems that superficial lesions are cured in 70–90% of cases but nodular lesions only in 60–80%.

Bowen's disease and solar keratosis have been treated satisfactorily with this drug, with success rates around 70–90%. There are few long-term data on recurrence rates.

15

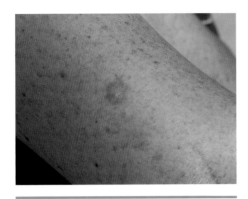

Basal cell carcinoma on the
forearm before treatment

Pale scar remaining at 1 year

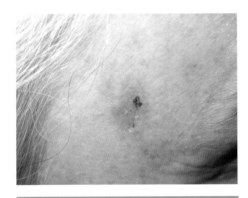

Basal cell carcinoma on the
temple

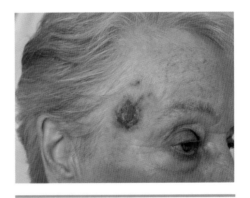

Area 8 weeks into treatment

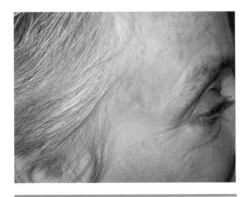

Area 12 weeks after finishing
treatment

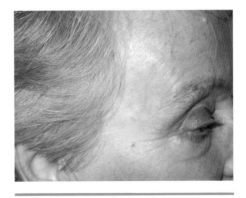

Area 1 year later

5-Fluorouracil

5-Fluorouracil is used to treat actinic keratosis, Bowen's disease and basal cell carcinoma. There is more than 30 years' experience with this drug. Despite its widespread use it has the drawback that it cannot penetrate through thick keratinized lesions. However, because it does not affect normal tissues it can be applied widely around the diseased area and it will deal with not only the visibly abnormal areas but also subclinically affected cells which become inflamed. The effect can be quite dramatic and patients need to be warned about this to ensure compliance with instructions.

Advantages

- Can be used to treat large areas
- All the abnormal cells in the treated area take up the drug
- Simple to apply at home
- Can be repeated numerous times over years

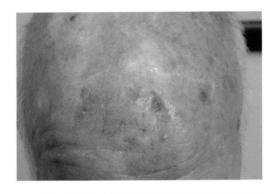

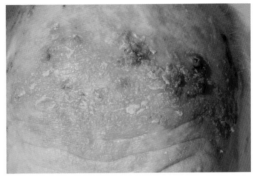

Lesions on the scalp before treatment   Area during treatment

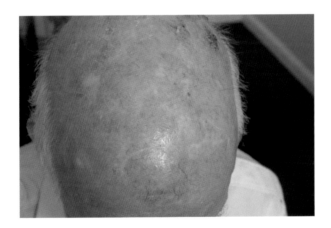

Area after treatment

5-Fluorouracil

5-Fluorouracil is used chiefly to treat solar keratosis and Bowen's disease. It is less effective for basal cell carcinoma.

There are many treatment regimens for 5-fluorouracil. Some doctors prefer continuous application on a daily basis until an inflamed response is achieved. If this does not occur within 2 weeks, then application is twice daily until the inflammation appears. Other experts recommend an intermittent approach (e.g. applying the cream daily for 1 week, then having 3 weeks off).

Disadvantages

- Cannot penetrate through thick lesions
- Does not penetrate to the base of hair follicles, etc.
- Usually produces a marked inflammation when it is effective
- Treatment may need to be repeated

Effectiveness

5-Fluorouracil cream is used in many countries but the strengths and preparations vary and so it is difficult to compare results. On the whole it is thought to be effective in treating the majority of thin solar keratoses but new lesions inevitably arise with time. Bowen's disease responds in 70–90% of cases, and superficial basal cell carcinomas may be successfully eradicated in up to 80% of cases.

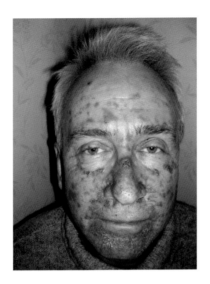

Marked reaction to 5-fluorouracil being used for
extensive solar damage

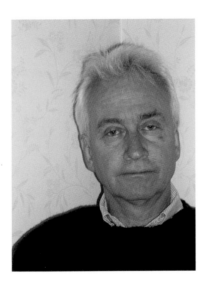

After treatment: slight redness, which gradually settled

With thanks to John Holmes, BBC Radio Nottingham, who gifted
these photographs of his treatment.

Photodynamic therapy

Photodynamic therapy is a technique which can destroy unwanted or diseased tissue whilst sparing normal tissue. First a drug called a photo-sensitizer is administered to the patient, either as a cream or by injection. The photosensitizer alone is harmless and has no effect on either healthy or abnormal tissue. However, when light (sometimes from a laser) is directed on to tissue containing the drug, the drug becomes activated and the tissue is rapidly destroyed, but only precisely where the light has been directed. Thus, by careful application of the light beam, the technique can be targeted selectively to the abnormal tissue.

Advantages

- Outpatient procedure
- Several lesions can be treated at one sitting
- Can be used for patients with fear of surgery, bleeding disorders, etc.
- May be good in areas of poor healing
- Generally excellent cosmetic outcome

Effectiveness

Results for superficial basal cell carcinoma are around 90% initial success but up to 10% of lesions recur over 3 years. Thin nodular lesions may respond in up to 90% of cases but recurrence is higher at around 14% at 4 years.

For Bowen's disease the currently reported overall initial clinical clearance rate is 90–100%, with recurrence rates of 0–11% in studies where follow-up has been for at least 12 months. The success for solar keratosis is similar, but judging recurrence in areas of extensive damage with multiple lesions is not easy.

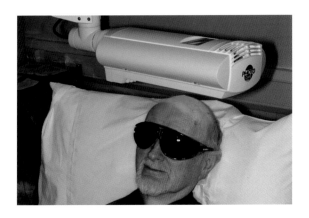

Red light being used for photodynamic therapy

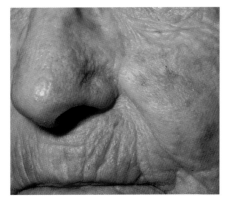

Actinic keratoses pretreatment

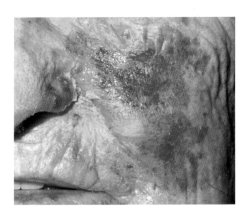

Post-treatment inflammation

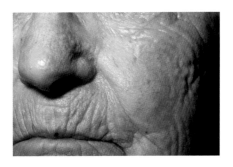

Keratoses cleared 3 months later

Photodynamic therapy

Progress

It is a rapidly developing field and there has been a shift to using methylaminolaevulinic acid (MAL), a more lipophilic methyl ester of 5-aminolaevulinic acid, in earlier use. As with all new treatments it is important to wait for the long-term follow-up studies before commenting on the overall benefit. However, it appears to be particularly useful for Bowen's disease and superficial basal cell carcinoma in poor healing sites and when the lesions are large, making other treatment options less attractive.

Disadvantages

- Painful – burning or stinging can be considerable
- Equipment and drugs are not cheap
- May require second treatment
- Not yet widely available

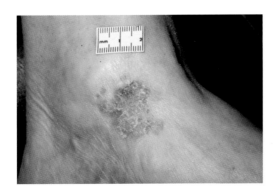

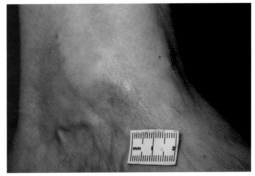

Bowen's disease

3 months after photodynamic therapy

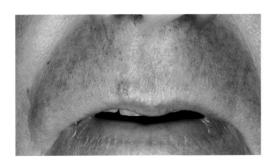

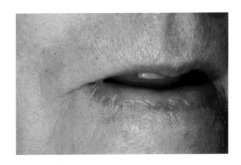

Basal cell carcinoma before treatment

3 months post photodynamic therapy

Index

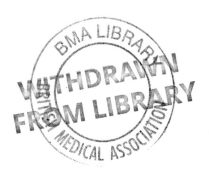